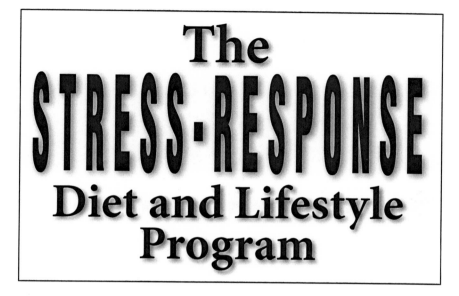

The STRESS-RESPONSE Diet and Lifestyle Program

A Hormone-Balancing Diet
and Exercise System
to Help You Achieve
Permanent Weight Loss,
Optimal Health, and Longevity

BILL CORTRIGHT

To order additional copies of this book, contact:
Xlibris Corporation
1-888-795-4274
www.Xlibris.com
Orders@Xlibris.com
60363

Contents

PART ONE

Understanding the Stress Response

PART TWO

The Body

PART THREE

The Mind

If you have health, you probably will be happy, and if you have health and happiness, you have all the wealth you need, even if it is not all you want.

—Elbert Hubbard

Endorsements

"If you are smart, you will listen to what Bill Cortright has to say. He is not speaking as one who has done his research in a library or through someone else's experience. He has been on the front lines for years, successfully helping thousands of people regain control of their health. If all you are interested in is getting sick, having surgery, and taking drugs, then don't read this book. But if you want to stay healthy and vital for your entire life, listen to this man. This is the real thing."

Frank Shallenberger, MD
Medical Director of the Nevada Center of Anti-Aging Medicine
Author of Bursting With Energy and The Type 2 Diabetes Breakthrough.
Editor of the Real Cures Newsletter

It was a great pleasure to review this new book written by Bill Cortright. In several occasions he has said to me: "I don't know much, I am not a Doctor . . . " However, it is thanks to the great understanding and with the experience of creating outstanding results for his clients that he has been able to draw such ground-breaking conclusions which he shares with us in this book.

His unique integrated concept of hormonal balance, stress response, proper diet and intelligent exercise will almost guarantee a happy and healthy longevity.

I am one of his many success stories. I have followed Bill's plan during the last nine months. It is not difficult at all, I look better and feel happier and healthier, more energetic. In just three months I gained 10 pounds of muscle mass and lost 14 pounds of fat; I feel like a new me. My most sincere congratulations and thanks for taking the time to write this book."

JORGE E. HIDALGO, M.D.
Director and founder of Juvencia Clinics of Plastic Surgery in Miami, Fl and Lima, Peru
Certified by the American Board of Plastic Surgery
President of the Peruvian Society of Antiaging Medicine and Longevity.

I have worked very closely with Bill for the past 5 years in promoting wellness medicine. In my years of practicing medicine in the US and in Panama I never encountered a person with more knowledge on how the body functions in regards to nutrition, exercise and stress as Bill has. It was really rewarding for my practice to finally find the link between the medical field and the fitness world. As physicians we are always recommending our patients to eat better and exercise without much feedback on whether what they were doing was right for them. With the Biofit center created by Bill, I was finally able to talk to somebody in the fitness world that fully understood how to blend these two fields together.

The results have been impressive. We have worked together with many patients that were following the wrong nutrition and exercise routine for them, and by evaluating them at a hormonal level we designed the correct nutrition, exercise and the right supplements that made remarkable positive results in these patients.

This book is the result of all this knowledge that Bill has acquired through all these years working in the medical and fitness fields.

I really feel that anybody who reads this book will greatly improve their ability to understand how the body works in regards to stress, exercise and nutrition to improve their quantity and quality of life.

Bill, it's been a true pleasure working with you.

Your friend,

Jorge Paz Rodriguez MD
Board Certified in Internal Medicine
Medical Director of Wellmed Clinic in Panama
Medical Director Stem Cell Institute
Email: Drpaz@cellmedicine.com

" . . . very direct, precise and down to the point. A very usefull tool in our quest towards maintaining a good lifestyle. Great resource to every person who wants to maintain a healthy mind and body. Definitely recommended."

Adriano Delgado, MD
Endocrinology and Metabolism
Physician Nutrition Specialist

"Bill's new book "The Stress Response Diet" is a complete guide towards a healthy and prolonged life. He has put into this book all the knowledge and experience that he has gathered since he was a small kid. He is a consummate professional and the best in his field.

I was very lucky to meet Bill at a time when I was diagnosed with heart problems, me being a Doctor I thought it was going to be easy to nurse myself into health but the more I read and asked among my colleagues what should I do? the more frustrated I got and the worse I felt. They told me I should loose 30 pounds, exercise more (I exercised 1 hour a day 5 X week already!!!) and go on a strict diet plus a bunch of medications to control my lipids.

When I first went into Bill's office and he started his examination, I immediately started noticing a way out off my problem and a change in my state of mind and lifestyle. What he recommended I did is all clearly explained in his new book. His book is a complete guide of what we should do to stay in shape and, like in my case, how to nurse ourselves back to health.

It has been more than 5 years since I've meet Bill and he has made a big change in my life and health, I can still, at age 50 enjoy the sport that I love so much, surfing."

Ernesto A. Calvo L., MD. S.A.A.O BC., S.A.C.S.

Acknowledgement

I would first like to thank the universal intelligence known as God, and the incredible daily guidance I receive from it in the pursuit of my purpose here on earth. Without this wonderful relationship I wouldn't have been able to achieve all that I have.

I would like to give a special thanks to my partner and my wife Hindy. If you had not come into my life I would have never found my way. Your love, faith and guidance mean everything to me.

I give a special "thank you" to my family. My children, Lexie, Chelsea, Natalia, Isabel and Brett. Your support over the years while I traveled the world doing research has been amazing. Your unconditional love gave me strength during the times when I had to be away from home.

I want to thank Henry and Margie for being there for me during the ups and downs of this and my many projects. You have truly been the best Mom and Dad I could ever hope for.

I would like to thank my team at BioFit, especially Javier for his outstanding work ethic, loyalty and for keeping the business growing while I was gone. I would also like to thank all the Doctors I have worked with over these years, especially Dr. William Evans, without his research I could have never created this program.

Dr. Jorge Paz Rodriguez, who has been a great partner in developing this wellness concept. Dr. Frank Shallenberger for providing the missing pieces of the program.

Dr. Adriano Delgado, for being the best Endocrinologist I have ever met, his view on wellness is priceless.

I have had the privilege to meet and work with many health professionals around the world; I thank you all for your contributions.

Finally, I give thanks to all my clients in Panama, Peru, United States and around the world. Without your believe in the Stress Response Diet I would not have completed this book. I thank everyone who has collaborated on this book from the testing, graphics, editing and publishing. It's been three years of hard work.

From the bottom of my heart I thank you all.

Foreword

Managing the Stress Response Is the Answer

One morning a few years ago, I was having breakfast with my daughter when she asked me, "Daddy, What do you do for a living?" Without thinking, I gave her my standard answer, "I help people to get healthy, lose weight, manage their stress, and create healthy lifestyles." As I looked up, I could see the puzzled look on her face; she didn't understand a word I had just said. I then replied, "Honey, our body works like a machine, and I fix broken machines."

Our bodies are like very complex machines with many interactive parts that must work together in harmony. If one element of our machine is not working well, then the entire machine seizes to function optimally. I have found, after twenty years of working with people and research, that the most important factor that affects our health, how we age, what illnesses we get, and even our body fat level is determined by how our bodies manage and respond to stress. Even though it is common knowledge that many things also influence these factors, such as genetic background, where you live, and what your family's health history is among others, how our lifestyle succeeds in controlling the effects of stress is the most powerful influence in our biology.

Let's take a look at, and, in the process, redefine what stress is. Stress is a physiological response for survival. Its job is to keep us alive through the fight-or-flight reaction. It is a primal and instinctive response built into our DNA through millions of years of evolution. It manifests itself in different ways, and here is where most people misunderstand stress. When you are angry or overwhelmed, you are consciously aware that you are under stress, but what most people do not know is that your body is under the same level of stress during less obvious circumstances.

For example, even though exercising is a positive activity for our health, if performed incorrectly or in extremes, it can be interpreted by your body as a stressor. When you are in a spinning class and you reach a level of high intensity performance, your body cannot tell if you are safely working out or being chased by a pack of wolves. The biological and physiological reaction in your body is the same in both circumstances. Your daily diet and the way your body processes different foods can also become a stress factor for your body because the chemical reaction produced by certain foods you eat alter the three key hormones that determine the way your body responds to stress. The key hormones that directly affect your body's stress response are adrenaline, cortisol, and insulin.

Adrenaline is produced by the adrenal gland. It stimulates the heart rate and dilates blood vessels. Adrenaline is naturally produced in high-stress or physically exhilarating situations. Cortisol is also secreted by the adrenal glands and involved in proper glucose metabolism, regulation of blood pressure, insulin release for blood sugar maintenance, immune functions, and the anti-inflammatory responses. Insulin is a hormone produced by the pancreas that regulates the level of glucose, which is a simple sugar that provides energy, in the blood. One could say cortisol and adrenaline break the body down while insulin helps to repair it.

The challenge we face in today's world is that we all live in a state of chronic stress, and we simply cannot shut off our body's stress response. This inability to regulate our key hormone levels through a balanced cycle of relaxation and activity affects the way our body does everything. Globalization, modern technology, easier and faster ways to travel, and all the high-speed, fast-food, instant-gratification comforts of modern living keep us constantly on the run and on the move. Modern life in its most "normal" form is stressful to our biological makeup.

This is why more stress-related illnesses are growing into epidemic proportions. More thirty-year-olds are having massive heart attacks, younger and younger children are suffering from morbid obesity, more women are entering menopause in their early forties, and younger people are suffering older-people diseases. These are all signs that the stress response is out of control and out to get us.

The stress-response diet program that I will share with you in this book is a new and innovative approach to many old problems. It is a program built on a hormone-balancing diet, supplement recommendations, and exercise routines that will help you create the lifestyle you need to counteract the damage done by your stress response. In this book, I will share with you the stories of many of the clients I have worked with for the last twenty years and how they were able to achieve optimal levels of health by understanding their body's stress-response signals and how to manage them.

I am grateful to have the opportunity to share with you what I have worked on for many decades, and I hope from the bottom of my heart that this book helps you to live a healthier, happier and more productive life.

Bill Cortright
Miami, Florida
2009

Introduction

A Quest for Self-Discovery

My personal journey with weight loss practically began at birth. I remember weighing close to 160 pounds at the age of ten. Growing up, I was one of the fattest kids in class. This caused me a lot of suffering, as I was under the constant barrage of bullying and teasing. I visited what seemed like countless number of doctors, nutritionists, and all sorts of other weight-loss experts in my quest to lose weight. To be quite honest, I remember those early years well, and the real problem was that I really didn't want to lose weight. My problem was that I loved to eat; food was like my best friend in those days.

What brought me to the point of obesity is actually a familiar story for my generation. My parents had gotten a divorce when I was young. This was common for many families in the late sixties and early seventies. I was young and had a terrible time making this adjustment. When it got to a point where I was too much to handle, I was shipped off to my grandparents to live with them. I found myself in a situation where I had started a brand-new life. I was in a new state, city, school; and everything that was familiar was gone.

Being raised away from my parents and siblings caused me to feel like a social outcast. I had trouble making friends and spent much of my time alone. The final blow to my childhood would come a couple of years later when my grandfather had a terrible industrial accident. This accident would leave my grandfather crippled for life. This would be the biggest loss of my life. My grandfather was my hero, my father, and my best friend. This accident would take away the one role model I had. After the accident, I had to practically raise myself since my grandmother had to take care of him and did her best for me (she was an amazing woman). At this time in my life,

I turned solely to food for comfort. I would eat when I was happy, when I was sad, it didn't really matter. Food became my new best friend.

I was around age nine when I visited my first so-called diet doctor. I didn't really understand what was going on, but my grandmother really tried to help me lose weight. She would prepare special meals for me, weigh all my food, and attempt to feed me healthy combinations. I remember those meals as if it was yesterday; I really hated being on that diet. I would wait until my grandparents went to bed and then sneak downstairs and literally raid the kitchen. Another one of my favorite rebellious escapades was to go to the dime store whenever I had extra change and I would buy candy (candy bars used to cost ten cents. Imagine). Once my grandmother took me to a nutritionist, who put me on a diet, and when I returned thirty days later, I had gained six pounds. These actions truly broke my grandma's heart.

The first time I would really begin to get serious about losing weight was when I turned 12 years old. I began to try everything possible. I went to medical professionals and tried everything from pills to meal-replacement shakes; I even received shots from one doctor (not a clue what the shot was). I began to try every diet that was available at the time—low-carbohydrate diets, juice diets, low-calorie diets, high-protein diets, grapefruit diet, etc. I even ordered magic gadgets that were supposed to transform my body. All of this, along with wraps to melt fat and dozens of exercise programs, to get me that beach body (plus the girl). I invested in so many promises of quick, painless weight loss that I actually lost count of all the different programs.

The results of these diets and other schemes were always the same. I would lose weight, and then before I knew it, I would gain all of it back, *plus a few extra pounds*. The only thing I truly lost on all of those weight loss programs was my confidence and self-esteem. During my diet years, I estimated that I lost over 750 pounds while gaining back even more. Each time I lost one hundred pounds, it would be an incredible achievement; but in the end, it was all the same. I would regain the weight and begin my next search for that new diet or pill.

Finding the Power

After spending more than a decade on the weight-loss roller coaster, my final ride would come as I entered my twenties. I was at the end of another diet cycle, which means I was in the process of gaining my weight back. I had gained back a hundred-plus pounds; I weighed over 270 pounds and was now wearing a tight size 48 pants (all at five feet six inches in height). I had been laid off my first real job as an adult. The stress of being unemployed and a life with zero direction was just too much. I began eating out of control and was drinking heavily on a daily basis. I then fell into a deep depression, and everything seemed hopeless.

My compulsive eating had completely deteriorated my life. I wouldn't leave my house for days while eating and drinking out of control. After several months of this behavior, I finally hit rock bottom. I was contemplating suicide when I received an absolute miracle that changed my life forever.

I stumbled upon a book that would set my life on a totally new course, a course I still follow today, twenty-five years later. The book was *The Power of Positive Thinking* by Norman Vincent Peale. I had read all the diet and exercise books in the market, but I had never read anything like this. I can safely say this one book is the reason I'm here with you today. I can also say it's the reason I never gained back my weight and became successful in my field and my endeavors. It changed the most important element when it comes to weight loss and health; it changed my attitude and how I viewed the world. This is more powerful than any diet or type of exercise. For the first time in my life, I discovered the personal power of *positive thinking.* Many years later, I would learn the power the mind actually had on the body's stress response.

I read the entire book in one day; I literally could not put it down. I felt a sense of empowerment and unbelievable hope, something I had never felt in the past. Then I simply *took action.* I started to move again; I would go out for leisurely walks. I started by going around the block. It didn't seem like much, but this was the first step of my new life and a lifestyle that I haven't stopped living for over twenty-five years now. I created a new state of mind; I believed I could do anything. I got rid of all the junk food I had been consuming and started eating sensibly. When it came to the exercise, that little walk around the block turned into two to three hours of walking daily! Over the next six months, I dropped over 125 pounds.

Along with the weight loss came a new attitude. In the past, I had lost weight, but never had changed my entire self-image. This time, I wasn't the fat person with the thin body; I was dynamic, outgoing, and extremely confident. Yes, I looked different, but the biggest difference was that I felt different. I have worked with thousands of people over the years, teaching them the truth about losing weight and getting healthy. I can tell you that when they get this feeling I'm describing—that extreme self-confidence, a sense of knowing they are changed from the inside—they will always get results. I will be giving you the tools to get this feeling; it's the key to any type of accomplishment, especially weight loss.

The Crossroads

On past diet programs, I had lost tremendous amounts of weight. After losing the weight, I always found myself asking the same question, "What now?" I was over one hundred pounds lighter, but I still had a flabby body with skin hanging, especially around my middle, and was still unsatisfied with the way I looked. I weighed 150 pounds at the time, my lowest weight since I was ten years old. Yet even at this low weight, I would never dare to take my shirt off in public. As I mentioned earlier, I wasn't the same person anymore. I was determined to create the body I had dreamed of. A beach body like Charles Atlas (all us baby boomers know who he is). I felt lost. Should I lose more weight? Do I diet harder? What should I eat now? More walking? These questions and many more were haunting me.

During this period of my life, I was going from one change to the next. I lost my weight, and I started to take steps to change my entire life by starting college. It was there where my career would begin to take shape, but not from my studies (I was actually studying police science at the time). It was when I met a classmate by the name of Dan. Dan was a competitive bodybuilder. I had never seen such a muscular human being in my life. Back in the early eighties, there wasn't an array of fitness magazines like today (especially in Central Wisconsin). Dan looked like something out of a science fiction movie (the first time I saw him, I thought he looked disgusting).

I approached my new classmate and asked, "How did you get muscles like that?" His reply was direct and simple. "I work out." Work out? I didn't have a clue what this meant or what it could actually do for me. The one thing I did know was I had to find out how a human could change their body to look like Dan's.

I made arrangements to meet Dan at the school gymnasium. The school was equipped with a full weight-training facility. During this time in my life, I was living in a little town in Wisconsin with a population of less than ten thousand people. I had never seen a gym or a real weight room. It wasn't like today where there is literally a health club on every corner; the closest public gym was probably two hundred miles away. My experience with weights was limited to my school physical education class and that was one of those old universal machines that all schools seemed to have at that time. What I remembered most about those gym classes was how hard I worked to avoid attending them. In school, I wasn't very athletic; I never even completed the physical fitness tests, and now I was getting ready to go and work out. I was so intrigued that I just had to go see what it was all about.

The next day when we arrived, I was completely in awe. I had never seen anything like the machines or the people that were in that room. Everyone there was screaming and straining while lifting incredible amounts of weight. It was a sight to behold. I have to say my first impulse was to get the heck out of there, but I had to see for myself what this guy Dan was all about.

Dan started training first with lighter weights, and then the weights would get heavier with each exercise he did. One thing I noticed was that not too many of the guys working out looked like Dan. Most of them were very big but also seemed very fat to me. Dan was so much more muscular and defined, and he trained completely different from the rest. Most of the guys were training with heavy weights but looked awkward while they lifted. They threw the barbell and dumbbells around while Dan was more methodical to his approach. Dan's training was on an entirely different plane. As he lifted weights, he literally was growing before my eyes. As he got bigger, his veins were sticking out, and every muscle was separated and defined. At that moment, in that dim-lighted, smelly room, with all that strange equipment, my life would change forever.

The next day, I started my own training program, learning the fundamentals from my new friend Dan. I have been training now for over twenty-five years, and I still remember that first workout like it was yesterday. I took to the weights like a fish takes to water. I was exhilarated with every training session I did. I visited that weight room daily, trying to learn everything I could from anyone who would teach me. I learned how to power lift to build my strength and muscle size. I learned about bodybuilding and the importance of a proper diet and supplements. I stopped dieting to lose weight and started dieting to gain muscle. I learned training techniques, split workouts, forced reps, drop sets, pyramid training, and so many other ways to increase my muscles. The only thing on my mind during those days was lifting weights and training (yes, the same guy who never completed a fitness test). I never missed a workout.

After just a mere three months of meticulous training, I could see incredible changes in the way my body looked. My legs grew very fast; I actually had trouble fitting into my pants. Along with the legs, my shoulders were visibly wider; my chest and arms were also much bigger. The transformation in those first months was nothing short of incredible. But by far, the biggest change I experienced was the flabby skin hanging off my abdomen. Anyone who has ever lost significant weight will tell you that the stomach area never seemed to get tighter, no matter how much weight you would lose.

To me, the change in my abdomen alone was kind of a miracle. I remember before I had dropped my weight. I would stand in the shower, and I was unable to see my feet if I was to look down—that's how big my stomach was. With this change, for the first time in my life, I could actually tuck my shirt into my pants. When you are overweight, it's a big deal when you can stop wearing oversized clothing that covers you like a tent.

In three short months, my life had completely changed. Everything was great until the day I weighed in. I hadn't weighed myself since I started the weight training. As I think back, I used to weigh in all the time, but I was so fixated on my training I just didn't do it. When I did step on the scale, I had gained thirty pounds. This sent a wave of panic through me that I can't even explain. How could this happen? I had done everything right, and I was gaining weight.

The Scale Is a Liar

With my new eating habits and exercise regimen, I was gaining weight like crazy. Since my first diet at age nine, my life was measured by what the scale read. When I was on a diet, I would weigh in anywhere from six to ten times a day. I was what I call a *scale-aholic; I was addicted to the scale.* My moods, in fact my entire disposition, was ruled by which way the needle fell on that box of numbers.

This sudden increase in my weight shocked me; I really thought I would lose weight with all the exercise. In the past, this would have sent me into full panic mode; but this time, it was different. First, I didn't think the same way I did in the past. I was a *positive thinker*, and I had made it a habit to look for the good. Because of this change, I didn't focus on the weight gain (in the past, I would have jumped off a building). I focused on how good I was really looking. I focused on the way my clothes were fitting. I focused on muscles I didn't even know I had three months earlier. I focused on how unbelievably good I felt!

During those days, I had no idea that muscle weighed more than fat or that muscle was the key to a strong metabolism. I had no idea what a body composition was. What I did know is I looked really different, and everyone noticed. I could see my new stomach, my new chest; more importantly, I felt different. I was not just learning the truth; I was living the truth. After spending more than a decade trying to lose weight, I learned that *the scale is a liar*. Throughout this book, I will discuss ways to measure your progress while becoming biologically fit. The way we measure weight loss may be the key to whether we create permanent weight loss or not.

All my life, doctors and other health professionals would tell me what I should weigh. They would give me a ridiculous goal of 140 pounds for my height. Truth be told, I weighed 140 pounds at age nine. What I have found over the years is that it's impossible to tell someone what their perfect weight is. Our weight really doesn't matter as much as our biomarkers and body composition (I will discuss this in detail later in this book). Even today's new body mass index (BMI) is flawed. According to my BMI, I'm actually obese even though I'm 11 percent body fat with a 7.8:1 ratio of muscle to fat. The truth is that the measurements that matter more than your overall weight and that best illustrate your state of health are your body composition and your measurements.

In my opinion, the scale is one of the reasons why so many diets fail. The scale would cause me to push my diets harder when I would hit a plateau and stop losing weight. The moment I restricted the diet more, a binge would set off, inevitably resulting in me gaining back all the weight—plus more. Back then, what truly saved me from sabotaging myself and gaining the weight back the last time I lost it was how I felt. I was confident, energetic, and had more self-esteem than ever before in my life. I believe strongly that the changes in the way I thought were the real reason I succeeded in keeping the weight off.

My Promise to You

My experiences during what I called my diet years are what gave me the foundation for everything I have accomplished today. When people come to my office and sit across my desk, I have empathy for them and their struggles. I know what it's like to sit on the other side of the desk, looking for answers and hope. As I write this book, I want you, the reader, to know that I understand what every single dieter has gone through and is going through. I have done a countless number of diets and weight-loss programs, all offering me the solution to my problem, only to be left disappointed time and time again.

I promise to share with you what I have worked on for the past twenty years. The stories and lives of those people I have worked with are the greatest way to explain how this program will change your life. I will share with you everything that I have learned during this time. I'm a recovering compulsive overeater and former obese person; therefore, I know the pain, and I know the struggle. Most of all I know that it can all be mastered, and changed.

I will *show* you how to manage your health in a fast-paced, stressed-out world. I will *motivate* you to make the necessary adjustments to truly create the changes you seek. I will share stories of clients and doctors I have worked with so you can relate to the challenges of others seeking answers. Finally, I will *inspire* you to succeed by teaching you how to create permanent new habits of health, habits that will become automatic and part of your individual lifestyle.

Together, I promise you, we can create the changes you want. I always say, "If I can do it, anyone can." I want to personally welcome you to the stress-response diet and lifestyle program.

How to Use This Book

In the stress-response diet and lifestyle program, I will give you a complete blueprint to help you make the changes you need to live better and to live longer. The program I share with you here is designed to fit into your individual lifestyle. This is essential for long-term success. In other words, you don't fit into the program; the program fits you as an individual. Most weight-loss programs are designed for you to fit into them. For instance, some of these popular mass marketed weight loss programs will say: "Buy our foods and you will lose weight" or "do not eat any of certain foods and you will lose weight". It's like finding a pair of shoes you love, but they're a size too small. The stress-response diet and lifestyle program fits into your lifestyle, nobody else's. I will teach you how to become BioFit (biologically fit) and how to stay BioFit even when you travel, through the holidays, and when you just can't get the right foods. Tailoring your program is the key.

While going through this book and creating your program, I will share with you what I have found over the years to work well with many clients. The purpose of this book is to give you a whole new perspective about how your body works and a new value system in regard to what it really means to be healthy. I have arranged this book in the order that I believe you should be introduced to this new concept.

- Part 1 is about understanding the stress response and how it affects your body's ability to produce energy. Stress exists in different forms. Some are more obvious than others. By recognizing what has the potential to stress the body, it is easier to manage the harmful effects that may arise.

- Part 2 is about the body and the science behind the stress-response diet program. Education is the key to taking charge of your body. You really need to understand why the program works. I have made this section easy to understand. In it, you will learn about the cycles of health that we all live through. The ten biomarkers that are key to longevity, metabolism, and health and the five bio-links that will be the base of your program.

- Part 3 introduces you to the mind, and I will share my very personal experiences in creating the mind part of the stress-response diet and lifestyle program. Part 3 also contains what I consider to be the most important element when someone is trying to create change in his or her life. In "The Mind" section, you will learn about the comfort zone and its relation to your habits. You will also learn about the testing periods you will face during crucial points in your new lifestyle program. I have found that when people understand how the mind works, success is inevitable. The stress-response lifestyle program really starts in the MIND!

- Part 4. In part four, Creating your lifestyle program, you will receive the guidelines to construct and put together the links of your new stress-response diet and lifestyle program. We will go through each bio-link and begin fitting them into your life. In this part, you will create your menu, tailored exercise program, and supplement regimen.

The stress-response diet and lifestyle program is designed to give you all the information you need to take control of your health and your biological aging process, as they are all important elements toward a lifetime of health and longevity.

Part One

Understanding the Stress Response

Chapter One

What is the stress response and how it affects your health.

Nothing changes until you do.

—unknown

Tom's Story

Tom was a thirty-five-year-old up-and-coming architect when I first met him three years ago. He worked with a large development company and had just been put in charge of several important projects that were being built around the world. Tom had to literally travel around the world for two hundred-plus days per year. When I first met Tom, he was in great shape with a good diet and regular exercise routine.

Three years later, Tom came back to the clinic to see me, and I could hardly believe my eyes. He had gained over forty pounds of weight that seemed to be distributed all around his waist. When I ran his labs, they showed elevated insulin and cortisol levels, along with increased cholesterol and sugar. Tom's composition test showed a ten-pound loss in lean body mass and thirty-two-pound increase in fat. He complained that he was always tired during the day, but couldn't fall asleep at night. Tom experienced insatiable cravings for carbohydrates, especially sweets. He stated his current stress levels were an eleven on a scale of one to ten. With all this, Tom attempted to stay on a reasonable diet, but failed often with late-night binges. His exercise program had become sporadic at best.

In the three years since I had last seen Tom, he had become a corporate success and a metabolic mess.

The tests confirmed that Tom's body was totally stressed out. I made two programs for him, one for when he was home and another for when he traveled. In each program, I gave him the proper combinations of food and supplements his body needed to maintain a proper stress-response balance. I also gave him the right arrangement of exercises for travel and at home to help his body to recuperate. An additional recommendation I made to Tom, which to me was very important, was to prescribe a spa regimen that included massages and steam to detoxify his body.

In three months, Tom dropped close to thirty pounds of weight and six inches from his waist. He was energetic, sleeping well, and able to work at a level he hadn't been able to achieve in years. The great thing about Tom's story is that he accomplished all this while still maintaining his travel schedule. Tom's responsibilities hadn't changed; he still lived a high-pressure and stressful life. What changed was the way Tom's body handled the stress response. With some simple lifestyle changes, Tom's body was no longer breaking down.

What Is the Stress Response?

If you were to ask me what is the one thing it takes to be healthy, to lose weight, and to prevent premature aging, the answer would be *stress management*. In fact, after twenty years of research and helping thousands of clients worldwide to lose weight and become healthy, *I believe that stress and our stress response is one of, if not the major cause of the obesity epidemic we currently see today.* We can blame the fast-food industry all we want; the truth is stress imbalance is the leading cause responsible for the sharp increase in obesity and obesity-related illnesses. The connection between stress and deteriorated health is widely ignored by the medical field and the weight-loss industry. Stress is not just a feeling of being overwhelmed or anxious. It is a strong physiological response that can throw off the basic biological balance of the entire body. The stress response is a powerful hormonal response that will determine whether your metabolism will burn fat or store fat at any given time. Managing this response is key to creating a lean, healthy body. The challenge here is that most people and health professionals don't really understand what stress is. What I have seen in my research is that managing the stress response is about *balancing three hormones; these hormones are cortisol, adrenaline, and insulin.*

Adrenaline is the stress hormone that gets your heart beating faster when you get excited or angry. Cortisol is the stress hormone that gives you heightened senses when you are working on a big project or are worried about something. Both of these stress hormones have the particular side effect that they can break the body down. Ironically, both of these stress hormones are also what I call your success hormones. Without a certain level of stress, you cannot have success. Highly successful people actually are able to reach this level of accomplishment due to the fact that they learn to function and manage stress better than other people.

Cortisol and adrenaline's side effects run the body down, but insulin, the third key hormone, is designed to help repair the body, hence the natural balance of nature at work. It doesn't matter how high a person's stress levels are, what truly *matters is if their lifestyle will allow the body to repair itself,* which means keeping the muscle and biomarkers healthy. I can have a client who has an eight level of stress on a scale of one to ten and, with a proper lifestyle program, can stay healthy and balanced, much like Tom did. On the other hand, I can have a client with a level three stress and, if their lifestyle isn't balanced, they can be unhealthy and breaking down.

True stress management is more than time management or goal setting; it's about keeping these hormones balanced. To do so, it's essential that we have some idea of what stress really is. Our stress response is part of our survival DNA, and it's built into our biology from millions of years of evolution. If a million years ago, you came across a saber-toothed tiger, you wouldn't have had the rational mind to say, "What a beautiful animal, let's take a picture" or "let's put him in a zoo." No, your stress hormones, cortisol and adrenaline, would be released into your body for you to take action to fight or flight. This response was a matter of life and death. This is the stress response. The challenge we face in today's world is that our body doesn't know that it's the year 2008 or 2010; it still believes that it lives in a cave, and there is a saber-toothed tiger behind the tree.

With this understanding of the stress response, let's take a look at what happens to our body in today's world. Let's say you are stuck in traffic and you are late for an appointment and you are upset. Your body will react to this stress the same way it would react to the tiger. Here is what takes place:

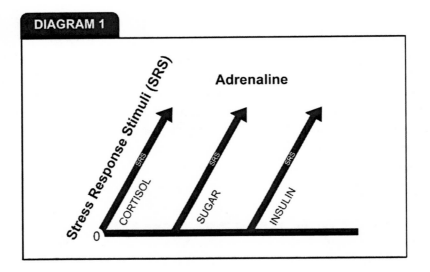

DIAGRAM 1

1. The body releases the stress hormones adrenaline and cortisol. The job of these hormones is to prepare the body to fight or flight. Your breathing will begin to increase, your blood pressure goes up, and your body prepares to take action.

2. The body needs a quick source of fuel so the cells can generate energy for you to take action. That fuel source is sugar. The question is this, "Where does the body get the sugar from?" The answer is we have sugar stored in our liver, and we have sugar stored in our muscles, but remember that our body holds a very limited supply of sugar. So what happens is this: cortisol goes to the muscle (biomarker one) and breaks it down into amino acids, takes those amino acids to the liver, and the liver produces sugar for the cells to create energy so we can fight or flight. This process is called gluconeogenesis. It basically is our body producing sugar without carbohydrates. I have treated clients who were on very low-carbohydrate diets that still showed elevated blood sugar levels much to their surprise due to this phenomenon. When gluconeogenesis takes place, it's a sign that our biomarkers are breaking down and also why stress can be considered the number one cause of aging, disease, and obesity.

3. After the body produces this sugar for "fuel," it needs to be driven into the cells so that we can get that quick energy we need for us to take action. To accomplish this, the body releases insulin. Insulin's job is to drive the nutrients into the cell so we can have energy to fight or flight.

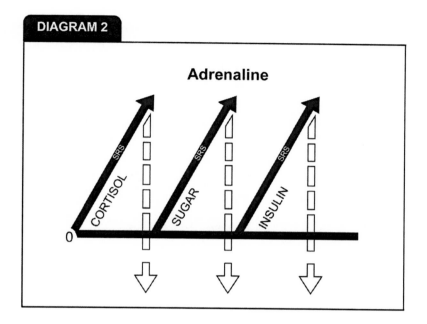

DIAGRAM 2

In diagram 2, you can see what happens after the stress response has taken place. What happens after we finally arrive to that appointment that we are late for because we were stuck in traffic? Well, the first thing that will happen is that your body is going to say, "This wasn't life threatening," and our stress hormones will drop.

1. After the stimulus, our cortisol drops down below its normal levels. Cortisol is our body's natural anti-inflammatory hormone. It is what protects us from inflammation. When we have low cortisol levels, we will lose our body's natural rhythm or balance. When we experience uncontrolled stress, the result is what some call metabolic burnout. The hormone cortisol is part of our body's natural rhythm. Cortisol rises in the morning to wake us up and prepares us for the day. It will increase our appetite and give us energy for the day's activities. At night, cortisol will drop, allowing growth hormone and melatonin to rise, helping you to sleep and repair your body for the next day. When we experience prolonged periods of stress, this natural rhythm will disappear. When I have clients that are burned-out, they will have very little appetite in the morning and during the day, but at night, they are literally starving.

2. Next, our sugar levels drop. Let's face the facts. When we are truly stressed out, we don't crave for a steak; *we crave chocolate ice cream*

(this is a communication). You are absolutely normal. Every time our sugar levels are too low, the commander in chief of the body, the brain, is going to demand that it is replenished.

3. Then our insulin levels drop low. Many health professionals believe that the lower the insulin levels are, the better. They couldn't be more wrong when it comes to the stress response. Insulin's job is to drive nutrients into the cell. If insulin is too low, the cell will starve, cease to function, and die. This is what is commonly known as aging. Every client I test with low insulin levels will also have a breakdown of muscle (biomarkers). It doesn't matter if the client is an executive or a professional athlete, they will have decreased biomarkers. Another characteristic common in most clients with low insulin levels is the fact that they usually have trouble sleeping at night. My theory is that low insulin leads to increased adrenaline. Adrenaline is what I call the alert stress hormone. This is the hormone that wakes you up right after you have fallen asleep, or it doesn't allow you to fall asleep at all. My simple explanation is this: our stress response is part of our survival instincts. If we are stressed all day long, our body perceives stress as life or death. So to protect us from our enemies, our body will keep us alert even if we want to sleep. It all comes down to our body's will to survive.

Today's Challenges with the Stress Response

The biggest challenge we face today is that we can never ever shut the stress response down. We can only manage it. Here are some sure signs that our stress response is out of balance:

1. You experience intense cravings for sweets and carbohydrates.
2. You are not hungry for breakfast but are starving at night.
3. You have trouble falling asleep or staying asleep.
4. You wake up feeling tired and unable to think clearly.
5. You feel stressed or overwhelmed.
6. You experience tachycardia (increased heart rate).
7. You cannot function without caffeine, especially in the morning.
8. You catch frequent colds.
9. You suffer from panic attacks.
10. You cannot lose weight. Even if you exercise more and eat less, your weight still goes up.

Most clients that I see, especially those older than thirty-five years of age, experience many of the symptoms of stress listed above. The biggest change I have seen in the last five years is the number of children I am seeing with these very symptoms. The reason is simple: their bodies are responding to too much *technology and chronic stress.*

Let's take a look at our modern-life working habits as an example. I am a baby boomer; the generation above me worked hard to build businesses. When they finished their workday, they would go home and unwind. In other words, they would rebalance the stress response. They didn't have cell phones, computers, e-mails, or televisions with five hundred channels. They actually rested for the next day. One of the key elements to balance the stress hormones is rest—that's when the body gets set for another day.

Now let's take the generation after us (baby boomers). They have been raised with technology. I have a twenty-one-year-old daughter who can take a computer apart and a seven-year-old son who can use a computer and play games on his Xbox without any help. The younger generations literally never shut off. They can be on the phone, working on the computer, and watching television all at the same time. With all this technology, they are consistently over-stimulated. This, coupled with being more sedentary, spells stressed-out! This will have a direct effect on their body's ability to manage the stress response. This is why today we see many children in their teens, and younger, suffering from metabolic syndrome and obesity.

My generation also has had tremendous challenges. When we went to school, we didn't even have calculators. We have had to change everything we know about surviving in today's business world. As a result, high-risk conditions such as heart disease and diabetes, which the generation before us would experience in their seventies, we are now experiencing in our forties and fifties. The media is looking for someone to blame—the fast-food industry, the schools, and even the parents. I have been working in this field for twenty-five years, and I am here to tell you that the major cause of obesity, disease, and premature aging is *unmanaged stress and an unbalanced stress response.*

Stress Response and Weight Loss

Maria was a forty-five-year-old stay-at-home mom with four teenage children. Maria weighed 378 pounds and was five feet six inches tall. She had been diagnosed with type 2 diabetes earlier that year. Maria sat in my office, desperate to find some way to lose her weight. Maria told me she started gaining weight at age twenty after having her first child; in fact, Maria told me when she was young, she could eat whatever she wanted and never gained an ounce. Maria's parents used to feed her extra food so she would gain weight as a child—a dramatic departure from how her adult life was unfolding. With each pregnancy, she would gain more and more weight.

Maria had tried several types of diets. Some were medically supervised, and others were the popular commercial diet programs. She had lost weight in the past, but every diet ended in the same way. She would be heavier than when she started. Maria lived a very active lifestyle, catering to all the kids' daily needs. She would rarely sit to eat her meals; most of them were on the run. When I took Maria through her initial evaluation, I actually found out she really didn't eat that much. It's a common misconception that people who are obese eat all day long. When I was at my heaviest weight, I actually was eating very little.

Maria's problem was not that she was overeating; her problem was she had an impaired metabolism. When we tested her body composition, her muscle to fat ratio was 1.3:1; a healthy woman would have a composition of 3.2:1 ratio. This meant that Maria's biomarkers were severely broken down. Bottom line, she had very little lean body mass.

I put Maria on the proper menu for her body and medical condition. I reviewed the menu with Maria's doctor for his approval. I tried to change his mind about letting her exercise, but he was adamant about losing the weight first. When she started, she weighed 378 pounds and was 43.4 percent body fat.

Maria adapted to the menu and her eating schedule with great ease. Every two weeks, she would come in for a follow-up appointment. She was losing weight very quickly, but she was complaining of increased fatigue and starting to have difficulty sleeping. After two months on the menu, we tested her composition again. Maria had lost exactly fifty pounds of weight. She now weighed 328 pounds. The problem was her body fat percentage was virtually the same, 43.2 percent. Maria had lost fifty pounds and NO FAT!

At the time, I didn't share these findings with her; she was really feeling tired and down, and when she saw how much weight she had lost, I didn't have the heart to bring her down. Within an hour, Maria's doctor called me to tell me how happy he was about her results. I told him these were terrible results; she wasn't burning fat at all. I again pleaded with him to let me start her on an exercise plan. I was again told no way until she weighed three hundred pounds.

Over the next thirty days, Maria lost another twenty-two pounds of weight. When we tested her composition, she weighed 306 pounds and was 43.4 percent body fat. This was the same exact body fat percentage she had when she started the diet, even though she was seventy-two pounds lighter. This is what happens with all diets. Maria's muscle-to-fat ratio (biomarkers) was exactly the same as it was before she started, a 1.3:1 ratio. The key to restoring our metabolism and health is by creating healthy biomarkers, not by necessarily losing weight.

When our stress response is out of balance, it becomes impossible to lose weight, especially to burn fat. There are several reasons why stress prevents any type of weight loss. Here are just a few:

1. When we are stressed out, we will have a change in our natural eating patterns. This is due to the unbalanced rythm our hormones are experiencing. When we are stressed out, our cortisol levels will be lower in the morning. We will not be hungry during the day and very hungry in the evening. This leads to what is called night eating syndrome, when your eating is heaviest at night and you have to eat large quantities of food to be satisfied. This makes it impossible to lose weight.

2. When we are stressed out, our sleep patterns will be disrupted. Without proper sleep, you cannot lose weight. When we are sleep deprived, our body goes into survival mode and wants to store more body fat in response to this signal of stress and sleep deprivation. Anytime the body perceives danger, it will store fat. Fat is its emergency fuel. The body will increase its hunger hormone, grehlin, and decrease its satiety hormone, leptin. Without sleep, the body cannot produce growth hormone, which is necessary for fat burning and health.

3. When we are stressed, we will crave for sweets. High-sugar foods will lead to increased insulin levels and literally shut off any attempt of the body to burn fat. When we eat these high-glycemic foods, this creates an insulin spike. The hormone that counterbalances insulin is cortisol. Therefore, each time insulin spikes, we inevitably produce more cortisol. In other words, by eating high-glycemic foods, you increase the stress hormones in your body.

4. In the part on "The Mind," you will learn that the subconscious mind is where our autonomic nervous system is located. This is what runs everything in our body. There are actually two parts of the

autonomic nervous system. One is the sympathetic nervous system, which is responsible for our stress response. This system's job is to prepare the body for danger by slowing down the metabolism and increasing fat storage. The other part of the autonomic nervous system is called the parasympathetic nervous system, which is responsible for our body's relaxation response and proper digestion of food, increasing our fat-burning response. How we manage our stress determines which stress response the body will turn on.

5. When our stress response is out of control, it will accelerate the breakdown effect on the ten biomarkers. This creates the domino effect, breaking down all the markers, starting with muscle. Less muscle equals a lower metabolism, which equals a lower aerobic capacity, which equals an increase in our fat stores.

The bottom line becomes very clear when we start to explore the facts of what it takes to burn fat and lose weight. Without proper stress management and controlling the stress response, you *cannot lose weight on diets alone*. In fact, most attempts at calorie-restrictive diets will end up making you gain extra weight. Being or gaining extra weight is only one of the issues. When we are stressed we tend to gain weight mainly around the middle and waist area, and this is the fat that increases inflammation in the body. Inflammation is the primary cause of heart disease, diabetes, aging, and Alzheimer's (we will discuss this further in the book). I believe that this imbalance in people's stress response mechanism has caused the obesity epidemic that we are currently seeing worldwide. The challenge we have is that society isn't going to slow down when it comes to technology and advancement. We have to teach proper stress management to thrive in today's world in order to be able to remain healthy.

Managing the Stress Response

Managing the stress response is about keeping the hormones balanced. This is accomplished with a proper lifestyle program. In part 4, "Creating your lifestyle Program," I will go into detail on the steps you need to follow to create the lifestyle program you need. For now, here is an outline of what I believe we need to focus on to better manage today's fast-paced world:

1. Proper diet. This may sound like a basic statement, but it's not what you think. When I refer to diet (as you will learn in the next

section), I'm referring to the right combinations of foods and snacks that will keep your body anabolic and fat burning. Diet is like taking medication when it comes to controlling the body's stress response. You must create a proper schedule for eating and put together the appropriate combinations of food for your particular metabolism. Eating the wrong foods at the wrong time can actually increase the stress response in the body.

2.   Exercise. Again, many will say this is common sense, but exercise has to be performed in a manner that will balance the stress response. If we exercise improperly (too much or too little), we will actually increase stress in the body, causing weight gain. Exercise as diet has to be tailored to the individual's cycle of health and lifestyle. *Now here's a fact: you cannot keep the stress response balanced, especially after age thirty-five without exercise.* Our bodies were not designed to be sedentary and under stress all day long. We need exercise to keep the body healthy. I will go into detail in the "Creating Your Lifestyle Program" section.

3.   Supplements. When it comes to supplements, most of the medical field has drawn the conclusion that it's nonsense. Supplements are just what they imply; they are meant to supplement your diet and give your body what it needs to be balanced. Like diet, supplementation is very individualized. The type and amount of supplements an individual needs is determined by the cycle of health, genetics, and current health status of the person. Supplements are not magic. Without the right exercise and diet, they will be ineffective. But with the right lifestyle program, they can make an incredible difference in one's health. In today's food supply, soil, air, and water are not the same quality they were as little as ten years ago; therefore, the food and produce supply in today's world has less nutrients and vitamins and other vital components. Couple this with today's incredible stress levels and it becomes clear that supplementation is a necessary factor to be healthy in today's world. The right type and dosage of supplements can literally make all the difference in a person's ability to manage the stress response.

4.   Testing. When we create a personalized nutrition and exercise program, we use a set of tests and blood test values to determine the health state and biological age of the client. These blood test values are based on our research after evaluating clients for two decades. In appendix A, you can see the blood test panel we look at and the

optimal values we use to evaluate how the client's body is handling the stress response. When we test individuals at the BioFit Centers (where we implement the BioFit program I created), we can take the guesswork out of their exercise and nutrition plans, each client needs to follow.

Thanks to this testing and evaluation system, we know the exact exercise program, diet, and supplements the individual will need to balance their stress response and lifestyle.

5. Water. I will go into this in detail in part 4, "Creating Your Lifestyle Program", where we discuss "Link Two: Hydration." Let me just make this statement: you can have the perfect diet and exercise program and still fail to balance the stress response if you don't drink enough water. When I work in corporations doing stress management, hydration is the first issue I will address.

The stress-response diet and lifestyle program will give you the guidelines that you need to truly cope with the stress of today's world. When you manage stress, you will manage your health. I have worked with thousands of clients and they have all achieved great results. I am sure you will find the answers you are looking for in this book. To get started in our journey, let's begin with the first thing we need to learn about and take control of: the body.

Part Two

The Body

Chapter Two

Starting with the Basics

As I see it every day you do one of two things: Build health or produce disease in yourself.

—*Adelle Davis*

When I first sit down with a client for a consultation, they always assume the answer to their health problems is to lose weight. Their doctor has told them that if they want to improve their health, they have to drop a couple of pounds. On top of that, they are bombarded with so many misconceptions about losing weight that most people do themselves more harm than good in their noble efforts to try to better their health.

My first assessment with a new client is about determining what their biological age is. Your true age is your biological age, not the number of candles on your birthday cake. Your biological age is dependent on how healthy your body is. It is measured by the ten biomarkers of aging (which we will discuss later in this book). The ten biomarkers are the base of the stress-response diet program and becoming BioFit. These markers not only determine if you're healthy, they are an absolute key to a strong and healthy metabolism.

Whether you are younger or older than your biological age, it depends on whether your body is *anabolic or catabolic*. When we are catabolic, it simply means our body is breaking down; we are out of balance. This usually means your hormones are out of balance. When we hear hormones, immediately we think sex hormones; but more often than not, it's your stress hormones that are breaking you down. When we are anabolic, we are balanced with a strong fat-burning metabolism; we are energetic and truly healthy. Our body is always going in one of these two directions; it never just stands still.

When I'm working with a client, the way their bodies communicate with them will often reveal a lot of information to me on whether they are anabolic or catabolic. At the BioFit Centers, I use a series of lab tests and other testing procedures to determine how a client's body is working. I will share with you these different procedures throughout the book. These tests will determine how the client's body is producing energy, and therefore, what their biological age is. You can be chronologically thirty years old and produce energy like a fifty-five-year-old, or you can be chronologically seventy and produce energy like a fifty-five-year-old. Both individuals are biologically fifty-five! So in order to help them get results, I have to treat both of them with the same program guidelines. It doesn't matter how old you are, it only matters how old you are biologically.

To create the stress-response diet and lifestyle program, I have worked with some of the top research scientists and doctors in this field. More importantly, I have been able to maintain my personal weight loss of one hundred-plus pounds for over twenty years by following my own program, so I guess that makes me living proof that it works. What I have discovered is that there are four elements needed to control the stress response and create permanent weight loss to create a biologically fit lifestyle, these are:

1. The mind. Understanding the workings of the mind is key in creating your BioFit body. Your mind influences your health on a moment-to-moment basis affecting the stress response.
2. The cycles of health. As we age, the body goes through distinct cycles. These are referred to as the cycles of health, and they will determine how your body will react to exercise and process food.
3. The ten biomarkers. These ten markers will determine whether your body is anabolic (balanced) or catabolic (breaking down). They will determine if your body is healthy at any given time. These markers will establish whether your metabolism is weak or strong. I use these ten markers when I am evaluating a client's progress, as they will always give me the true story of how the client is progressing.
4. The five bio-links: The five links are the base of the stress-response diet. They will give you the guidelines you need to live the BioFit lifestyle every day. These links work together to create a chain of health.

Introduction to the Cycles of Health

The body manifests common characteristics in four specific age groups that I have named cycles of health. The stress response affects these cycles in different and specific ways. When we begin to reach a certain cycle, the body changes the way it processes food and reacts to exercise. This means that you can have a perfect lifestyle program one year, and it will need to be modified the next because your body has changed. The four cycles of health are:

1. Twenty years and younger to age thirty-five.
2. Thirty-five to forty-five years of age
3. Forty-five to fifty-five years of age
4. Fifty-five years and older

Within each of these cycles, there is a distinct protocol to individualize your stress-response diet program. You can have the perfect diet and exercise program at age thirty, and the same program will not work for you at age thirty-five. The main key that I have found to create true weight loss, health, and longevity is to have each individual's program match how their body is working during the particular cycle they are in. *The cycles of health must be considered when developing any type of lifestyle program.* I will discuss these cycles in detail later in this book.

Introduction to The Ten Biomarkers

The ten biomarkers are key elements in the stress response diet & lifestyle program. Since the beginning of time, people have been fascinated by the quest to defy the aging process. Cultures across the world have contributed folktales about the fountain of youth and perfect utopias where people never age. The human race has always dreamt of winning the battle against losing its youth, vitality, and ability to enjoy living.

Modern science, although at its beginning stages of deciphering the mystery of aging, has evolved immensely in this field. Anti-aging medicine is becoming a big business and much of the time flies in the face of traditional medicine. One of the early Pioneers in the research of aging and health and fitness was Dr William Evans. Dr. Evans, along with his colleague Dr. Irwin Rosenberg in the late 1980s and early nineties, created the ten biomarkers from their research at Tufts University. The word *biomarkers* stands for "the biological markers of age." The ten biomarkers specifically describe the ten variables that make up aging and the sequence at which they may appear throughout an individual's life. By doing so, they provided a measuring tool to establish your biological age.

Dr. Evans and his research have been an instrumental part in my work to create the stress-response diet and lifestyle program. His research helped shape a lot of the basic criteria I use to work with clients. It gave me the answers to how our metabolism is influenced by aging or the breakdown of the body. The ten biomarkers are the markers I work to balance in order to help my clients achieve permanent weight loss and also how to reverse and prevent lifestyle related diseases such as diabetes and heart disease. I have used these biomarkers as a guideline for my work for the past twenty years. I will go into detail on all the biomarkers later in this book.

The ten biomarkers are as follows:

1. muscle mass
2. strength
3. basal metabolic rate
4. body fat
5. aerobic capacity
6. blood pressure
7. blood sugar tolerance
8. cholesterol
9. bone density
10. body temperature regulation

These biomarkers are the key to creating health, longevity, and permanent weight loss. These markers also determine if the stress response is balanced. When these biomarkers are broken down, they will create a domino affect on our health.

Introduction to The Five Bio-Links

The five bio-links are the foundation of the stress-response diet and lifestyle program. When the five links are practiced together, they create a strong fat-burning metabolism and an overall increased state of health. The bio-links give you a distinct blueprint to help you build a BioFit lifestyle and manage the stress response.

Below you will find a short description of each link. The bio-links will be explained further and be tailored for your individual program later in this book.

Link One
Meals

"You've got to eat to lose."

Link one explains the body's survival mechanisms and how you cannot force your body to change through restrictive diets. *Dieting has a direct effect on the stress response.* Link one explains why diets alone don't work and how it's not about willpower, whether or not you lose weight. You will be educated on the fat set point and how, by controlling it, permanent weight loss is attainable. In this link, you will learn how to change and control your metabolism by providing your body with specific combinations of foods at certain times in order to control the body's leptin levels and other specific fat-releasing hormones. (Leptin is a hormone that controls the release of fat from the fat cell in order to use it as fuel.) Most importantly, the diet you eat will always affect the stress response.

Link Two
Hydration

"You've got to drink to shrink."

Link two highlights the importance of drinking enough water to stimulate your body to get rid of excess fat and toxins while regulating the body's temperature. Most people know it is important to drink enough water, yet very few understand the physiological reasons for doing so. Link two also explains the effect of water on the body, the approximate amounts that men and women need, and how to tell if you are truly hydrated or not. Maintaining a proper state of hydration is essential to control the stress response.

Link Three
Circulation

"Know your zone to burn fat."

Link three explains the difference between aerobic and cardiovascular exercise. In this link, you will be educated on the changes of exercise intensity as we progress through the different cycles of health. You will learn how to take the guesswork out of your exercise by understanding the importance of working out smarter by monitoring your individual heart rate. Here you will learn how, by exercising too much, you can actually increase your biological age along with your body fat by unbalancing the stress response in the body. Link three gives you the answers to create a perfect exercise zone in order to get optimal fat burning at a cellular level. When you perform proper aerobic exercise, you can get results at any age.

Link Four
Lean Body Mass

"The key to metabolism and longevity."

Link four is a piece of the exercise puzzle that is often overlooked. In link four, lean body mass, it is about incorporating resistance training into our lifestyle. This link is the key to reversing our biological age and increasing our metabolism. I will go as far as to say that after two decades of helping people to lose weight, without this link, it's impossible to maintain any type of weight loss and overall well-being. You will learn how easy it is to fit these simple exercises into your individual routine. This link is the *key to longevity* and can be done no matter what age or current state of health. The stress-response diet and lifestyle program will give you the key and easy solutions to maintaining healthy biomarkers.

Link Five
Junk Night

"Have your cake and *eat it too!*"

Link five is a very important link to creating a lifestyle program that will last for the rest of your life. In this link, you will learn why it is essential to take a day off from your menu to keep the fat-burning hormones balanced. What science has learned recently is that our fat cells release hormones that determine whether you burn fat or you don't. The key player appears to be the leptin hormone. Link five helps to keep this hormone balanced, which allows for optimal fat burning. Junk night is also essential to give our bodies the correct communication to lower our fat thermostat (fat set point) so we can establish permanent weight loss. Basically, you have to cheat to win the fat loss game. Link five is also the psychological key to maintaining a new lifestyle program, it's six days on and one day off, so we reward ourselves once every week with our favorite foods. For managing the stress response, this link is as important as any.

Chapter Three

Introduction to The Stress-Response Diet and Lifestyle Program:

"The significance of a man is not in what he attains but in what he longs to attain"

—*Kahlil Gibran*

Why Diets Alone Don't Work

For you to create permanent weight loss, reverse the aging process, and lower your biological age, it is essential that you never go on another crazy, calorie-restrictive diet again. The stress-response diet and lifestyle program is not "a diet," as conceived by popular criteria because it is presented within the context of a lifestyle program; therefore, it is a way of life to create fat-burning metabolisms, optimal health, and longevity.

In fact, the meaning of the word *diet* according to the *Webster's New World Dictionary* is "one's usual food or special food taken as for health".

The goal of this program is not just to help you lose excess body fat, but to help you not to gain it back. Most popular (wrongly called) diets and food programs may be able to help you lose weight, but that's not good enough if you want to improve your health. The key to having the right nutrition plan is to have that plan fit your body's health needs while it helps you manage your stress response.

Elizabeth's Story

"I'm eating less and less food, and I'm actually gaining weight!"

Elizabeth, a thirty-eight-year-old business executive and mother of two, came to see me out of complete frustration. She complained, "I'm eating less and less food, and I'm actually gaining weight." Elizabeth continued, "I weighed between 112 and 116 pounds my entire life until four years ago. I now weigh 145 pounds, and I went up twenty pounds just this last year. It seems the harder I try to lose weight, the worse I get."

I understood exactly what Elizabeth was going through. I have heard this same story hundreds of times, especially those female clients of mine past thirty-five years of age. I personally knew that frustration of doing everything right, being disciplined, and mustering enormous willpower only to continue to gain weight.

The first thing I did with Elizabeth was to ask her about her personal health history along with a complete family history of any diseases. The first thing that came to my attention was that she had a hysterectomy at age thirty-five. At that time, she was diagnosed with polycystic ovary syndrome (PCOS) and had many cysts develop in her uterus. Elizabeth also had a strong family history of type 2 diabetes on both sides of the family.

When I examined Elizabeth's lifestyle, she explained that she was following a one-thousand-calorie diet that was very low in fat, which she received from her nutritionist. She wasn't doing any exercise at this time because she said she just doesn't have the energy to work out. Elizabeth also complained of having trouble sleeping and a strong craving for sweets. But she stated she didn't give in to the cravings, but sometimes would try to go to bed at 7:00 p.m. just to avoid eating.

As Elizabeth sat in my office, I could feel her desperation. Not only was she suffering, her family was also suffering. She was depressed, tired, and still gaining weight. I knew what Elizabeth's body was communicating. It was screaming, "I'm out of balance, and I'm trying to survive."

My first step was to contact Elizabeth's physician to see if I could request some blood tests. Sure enough, when her labs returned, her doctor confirmed what I had suspected. She had elevated insulin levels (a key hormone in managing the stress response), elevated triglycerides along with borderline high glucose levels. In fact, Elizabeth's triglycerides were over 400 mg/dl (optimal levels should be below 100 mg/dl*1). Elizabeth wasn't diabetic (yet), but she was very much insulin resistant. This meant the current diet she was prescribed was totally wrong for the way her body was functioning.

The next step was to get her body composition and determine her muscle-to-fat ratio. This ratio gives me an indication of how healthy her biomarkers are. A healthy woman with healthy biomarkers would have at least 3.2:1 ratio of muscle to fat. Elizabeth's test came in at a 1.8:1 ratio, showing a significant breakdown of the biomarkers. After getting her ratios, I proceeded to test her resting metabolic rate (RMR). This is the amount of calories the body burns at rest. Elizabeth's rate was low for a woman her age, it tested at 1,300 calories; but when I calculated her diet, she was only consuming 800 calories daily.

What was happening to Elizabeth is what happens to all of us when we go on a restricted calorie diet. Our body literally rebels and starts storing more and more fat (I will explain this in detail later in the book). The other problem was that her nutritionist gave Elizabeth the typical low-fat, food-pyramid-type diet. This particular diet was making her a metabolic mess. Elizabeth's body didn't process carbohydrates properly; her diet was composed of 70 percent carbohydrates with very little fat or calories.

Our plan for Elizabeth was to tailor her diet to the way her body was processing food and create an exercise plan that would help her body to begin burning fat at a cellular level. Within four months, she was wearing clothes she hadn't been able to fit in for ten years. More important than her dropping sizes was her laboratory results. Her triglyceride level dropped to 80 mg/dl and insulin levels were at optimal levels. In fact, all her tests were optimal, and she did it without any medication. Elizabeth also had an amazing body composition change; her muscle-to-fat ratio went to 2.8:1 and her body fat dropped from 36 percent to 26 percent.

Elizabeth's story is a daily occurrence at the BioFit Centers. With today's mass media and the various diet options they present, it becomes extremely confusing when it comes to choosing the right one. On one end of the spectrum, you have the experts telling you "don't eat any fat." On the other

---

*1. *Even though the American Heart Association considers triglyceride levels below 150 mg/dl to be at the normal range and low-risk levels, I have found that when people maintain triglyceride levels at 100 mg/dl or below there is an increase in their HDL cholesterol level greatly improving their lipid profile.*

side, you hear "eliminate carbohydrates completely." In the end, neither extreme is the answer.

As we age, our cycle of health changes; our bodies become more insulin resistant, which means we have more trouble processing carbohydrates. A diet that worked last year may be wrong this year. The bottom line is as you age, if you eat as the food pyramid recommends, you will soon look like the food pyramid!

Other diets that have been popular in recent years are the opposite of the pyramid. These are low-carbohydrate diets. These diets will also lead you to a dead end, as you will learn later on the carbohydrate section of this book. Every week, it seems that a new crazy diet comes out, and we rush out to get the next miracle weight-loss program.

Last year, people in the United States alone spent over $35 billion on different weight-loss programs. Now let me ask you, if those programs worked and the $35 billion bought answers and results, what would be this year's sales projection for the weight-loss industry? Well, you would naturally think that it would be less; but no, the projection for the next year is higher.

The bottom line is that the weight-loss industry gives you just what it promises, and that is plain and simple weight loss. Every one of those programs out there is geared for you to "lose weight" and not necessarily fat. *The stress response diet goal is not just to lose weight; it's to lose all excess FAT.* I know you're saying to yourself it's common sense. Yeah, yeah, Bill, I want to lose fat. But how does the diet industry measure your progress? By how many pounds you've lost. How do most doctors measure your health? By how much you weigh. Neither of these matter all that much; the true measurement is your body composition and the muscle-to-fat ratio. If I put you on a program and I drop twenty pounds off you, and those twenty pounds happen to be muscle, what have I just done to you? Well, I have just accelerated your aging process and destroyed your metabolism, plus you will probably gain quite a few extra pounds to top it all off. *Diets alone don't work!*

In this book, I will go over the body's will to survive and how it affects the stress response and how we control our body fat levels (weight). These distinct survival mechanisms are the reasons diets fail; they are also the keys to creating *permanent weight loss.* When we live a BioFit lifestyle, we produce lifelong results, working with our bodies instead of against them. The stress-response diet and lifestyle program will teach you the truth on how to become BioFit.

So what is the Answer?

Your body is an amazing self-adjusting machine designed for survival under the most extreme conditions. The answer to achieving optimal health and weight loss is to work with our body and give it the proper signals it needs to burn fat. By doing so, we will enjoy incredible energy levels and we will prevent any type of breakdown. We have to learn to listen to our machine when it tells us something is out of whack; like when your car's engine begins to knock or your oil light comes on, our body does give us similar signals when the stress response is off.

In Elizabeth Case, which I shared earlier in the book, her body was screaming out information. First, she was craving sweets, suffering from fatigue, hungry late at night, and was unable to sleep. Second, her medical history was telling us she had PCOS that will make the body have trouble with carbohydrates. Third, she had a strong family history of diabetes. If Elizabeth was a car, we would head straight to the mechanic. Unfortunately, most of us think it's normal to be tired, gain weight, and have our machine break down as we age. It's absolutely not true; our machine can run at an optimal level for our entire life.

The answer is to educate yourself on how your body is communicating its message to you. Are you tired even though you sleep? Do you exercise and still seem to be gaining weight? Does it feel like you're literally starving and your clothes are tighter? Are you more anxious, especially when it comes to food? Are you depressed, craving, ready to just give up? These are just a few of the body's signals that can give you a clue when setting your personal lifestyle plan. I will educate you through this book on how our body sends you signals when following a proper plan, plus how simple blood tests can reveal messages on how your body is working. Simply put, the stress response can be measured. These measurements are not as complicated as you think.

I have given you a brief introduction on how our body communicates key variables to us, a big part of balancing the stress response is also how we communicate with our bodies. "The Mind" section in this book is probably my biggest secret for maintaining my weight loss. I will teach you how to create the body and health you want by stopping fat thoughts and creating new permanent lifestyle habits. After years of working with clients and keeping detailed records, I realized a distinct pattern that took place when anyone was changing their lifestyle. I could tell when a client would begin to self-sabotage their program. I will teach you when these testing periods will appear and simple techniques to help you smash through them.

The objective of this book is to educate, motivate, and inspire you to make the changes that will set you free from restrictive diets, crazy exercise, and short-term fixes that leave you frustrated and worse off than before you began the program. My promise to you is that when you control the stress response and become biologically fit, you will lose your weight and increase your health, all while decreasing your biological age. You will get all this without hunger, cravings, and pain.

The secret is to balance our body for optimal energy production. Simply, we need to program our body to burn fat. I will share with you the ten reasons your body doesn't burn fat and give you the keys to unlock your body's fat-burning potential. Another secret to permanent weight loss and health is reprogramming your mind so your body knows that its metabolism is strong and that illness is not an option in your life. I will discuss later on what I believe is the true cause of the obesity epidemic (and it's not fast-food restaurants).

I would personally like to welcome you to the stress-response diet program and to your new biologically fit body. Please enjoy the journey and the results.

Chapter Four

Understanding The Cycles of Health

"Everything in life goes in cycles and everything has its turn. Everything moves on and grows, evolves and changes. Nothing lives on that stagnates . . ."

—Margo Kirtikar

Slowing Down of a Champion Tri-athlete

Don was a thirty-seven-year-old champion tri-athlete and was one of the top-ranked athletes in the area. Don had competed in these grueling events for over fifteen years. When I met Don, he was thoroughly depressed and completely run-down. He was complaining of fatigue, but couldn't sleep at night (unbalanced stress response). He stated that for the first time in his life, he didn't feel like competing or training. Don was also disheartened by his last few competitions as his times were falling as fast as his energy levels were. He did tell me he was having trouble with his training because of frequent injuries and fatigue.

The first thing I established with Don was, did he really want to continue competing, as I explained that being a tri-athlete isn't the healthiest sport in the world. He assured me that he had no intentions of retiring anytime soon. I then started testing Don to see what was going on. I sent him to a doctor to have his hormones checked, to see if there was an imbalance. I then put him through the BioFit cardio-metabolic stress test called the bio-energy test. This would show me how Don was producing energy and what his optimal aerobic training zones were. Finally, I did a body composition test, which would give me his muscle-to-fat ratios and determine how healthy his biomarkers were.

When I received the tests, I was quite amazed at the results. First, Don's biomarkers were diminished. His muscle-to-fat ratio was 4.2:1. The ratio for a healthy male is 5.2:1, and the proper ratio for Don's sport would be 6.5-7:1. This explained why he was getting injured; he didn't have the muscle to protect his joints. During his cardio-metabolic stress test, (bio-energy), we could see a quick rise in carbon monoxide, which gave me the indication that he wasn't using fat for energy. This would be the reason Don was experiencing low endurance and fatigue. Finally, I received the hormone tests, and his total and free testosterones were both low. These tests gave me the answers to Don's problems.

The first thing I did with Don was to really get his diet balanced so he could recuperate from his training. I then gave him the proper supplements to allow his hormones to balance naturally. The cardio-metabolic stress test gave him the precise exercise zones for his training. We also added resistance training to his exercise regimen. This was the first time Don had to pay so much attention to diet, supplementation, and exact heart rate zones in all his years of training.

The results were incredible. Within thirty days, Don's muscle-to-fat ratio improved dramatically, along with a dramatic increase in energy, and the injuries disappeared. Don returned to his championship form and went on to win his next race.

What happened to Don was simple. He got older. It happens to all of us, and you don't have to be an athlete to experience a decline in performance. When we experience fatigue during the day, but cannot fall asleep at night. When we start to lose concentration and start to forget more we need to realize that our body is sending us a message. The lifestyle that worked at age thirty doesn't work any longer at age thirty-five. These are the cycles of health and the stress response.

The different age groups that I have worked with over the last twenty-five years have ranged from eight years of age all the way to ninety-three years of age. In the beginning, I worked with a more athletic younger crowd, ranging from twenties to early thirties. I then worked with children, setting up nutrition and exercise programs for schools. In the mid nineties, I focused on corporations and executive wellness, ages into the mid-fifties. Finally, the last years before I started the BioFit Centers, my average-age client was seventy years of age. I was one of the first to work with seventy-, eighty-, and ninety-year-olds. With all this experience of working with different ages, I created the cycles of health. The four cycles are:

1. Cycle one: twenty years and younger to thirty-five years of age
2. Cycle two: thirty-five to forty-five years of age
3. Cycle three: forty-five to fifty-five years of age
4. Cycle four: fifty-five years and older

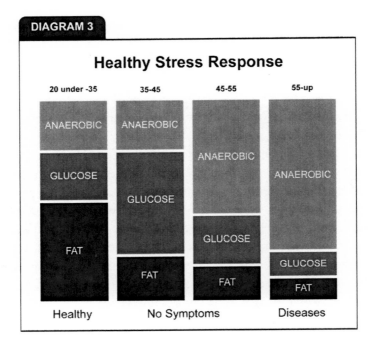

During these cycles, the body will change the way it produces energy. (Refer to diagram 3, healthy stress response). In cycle one, we are young and healthy and our body uses mainly fat to create energy. In cycle two, we start to use less fat and more glucose to create energy. This creates an energy deficit that I will go into detail later in the BioFit cell. In cycle three, we start producing energy more anaerobically (without oxygen) and our biomarkers start to break down. In both cycles two and three, we are not displaying signs of illness; in fact, we may feel fine. Finally, in cycle four, we now produce all our energy from anaerobic energy, this is when we get sick and start needing medication.

Our chronological age is not the only variable that determines our cycle of health. Our personal energy cycle is what actually determines what cycle we are living in and what our *biological age is.* You can be chronologically thirty years of age and produce energy like a fifty-five-year-old, and you would be biologically fifty-five years. On the other hand, you can be seventy years in the chronological age and produce energy like a thirty-year-old.

You would biologically be thirty. It doesn't matter how old you are, what matters is how old you are biologically. At the BioFit Centers, we use a quick cardio-metabolic stress test, also called bio-energy test, to determine the biological age of our clients by measuring how their bodies are producing energy. We can keep our body in cycle one at any age if we can remain balanced. Let's take a look at the changes we experience in each cycle.

Cycle One
Twenty Years and Younger to Thirty-five Years of Age

In this cycle, the body can take a tremendous amount of abuse. We don't have to eat right, exercise much, and can get by with little sleep. Under normal circumstances, the body can be pushed hard. This is also our athletic cycle when we can take our bodies to the limit to see what we can do. It's time when most of us will throw caution to the wind and live a little bit on the wild side.

When it comes to dieting, this is definitely the weight-loss cycle. This is when you can eat whatever you want, and then with a couple of days on the diet of the month, you can drop the weight without any problem. It's also a time when the "no pain, no gain" exercise philosophy of aerobics classes, spinning, and boot camp training can work for fast weight loss. This is our athletic cycle when we can train for sports and athletic events, and the body can recuperate without much problem.

When I see clients in this age-group, they are worried only about losing weight and not too much about their health. In most cases, they are healthy and not in need for any medications. In the BioFit Center, this group only compromises about 10 percent of the clients. In normal fitness centers, this cycle is the main age-group that makes up its membership. This group will begin to notice subtle changes as they hit thirty-two to thirty-three years of age, which is when they begin to enter health cycle two.

Cycle Two
Thirty-five to Forty-five Years of Age

In the second cycle of health, everything will begin to change. The diet and exercise program or the lifestyle you lived in the first cycle no longer works. In this cycle, you start to experience more fatigue and weight gain. Dieting is no longer much of an option as it becomes more difficult to lose your excess weight, and people begin to feel too tired to sustain their previous type of exercise regimen. Most people will tell you "when I hit forty, everything changed." What they don't understand is the change began at age thirty-five, but they started to notice it at age forty.

What changes in the second cycle? The body no longer handles stress the same way it did in the first cycle. In other words, if you were faced with a certain a problem or stressful situation at age twenty-five, you would deal with it and move on quickly without many consequences. But if you are faced with the same exact situation at age thirty-five, you will most likely address the issue in a similar manner as you did ten years earlier, but it will take much longer for your body to recuperate from the stimulus. When we are talking about the stress response, it's not just the mental stress we are talking about, it's the way the body physically handles stress. It's about managing our body's stress hormones and the stress response. We start using less fat and more sugar to create energy, thus creating an imbalance of energy in our body. You start gaining weight, especially around the middle and may seem you're always fatigued.

When I see clients that are in the second cycle of health, they are not as concerned about weight loss any longer, they *want to feel better*! Many of these clients are now starting to take medications or have been told by their doctors that they are borderline diabetics or reaching chronic high blood pressure or beginning to see the physiological signs of some type of chronic stress in their bodies. These clients feel stressed out, overwhelmed, and are having trouble sleeping, along with the added weight gain. When they go to the doctor and explain their symptoms, they are told nothing is wrong with them—they're just getting older. But there is something wrong; it just can't be measured with conventional medical testing. What has changed in this cycle is the way the body handles stress and the way it is producing energy. The body is using less fat and more sugar for energy production resulting in less consistent levels of mental and physical energy, more cravings, and weight gain.

I have found that clients in the second cycle of health no longer benefit from extreme exercise and restricted calorie diets. The body in the second cycle has to be fed with the proper combinations of foods at the right times to maintain a proper balance of the stress response. Unlike the first cycle, if you do not eat properly, your body cannot function at a very high level for long. To maintain athletic competition in the second cycle, the diet has to be perfectly balanced with the training. In Don's case, for him to be competitive in his sport, he had to maintain an ideal balance between diet, training, supplements, and rest.

In cycle two, our lifestyle must change in order to promote health and wellness in our body. Diets will no longer work, and our goals will become more about health than weight loss. What's great about the second cycle is that when you start focusing on being well, you will automatically lose weight. At the BioFit Centers, the percentage of clients that make up the second cycle is over 30 percent. Over the years, we have run thousands of tests on our clients in this cycle and the stress-response diet protocols will easily help you create a balanced lifestyle that will allow you to achieve all of your goals.

Cycle Three
Forty-five to Fifty-five Years of Age

In the third cycle of health, the body will accelerate its breakdown. Once again, everything that worked in the second cycle no longer works in the third. The diet and exercise regimen that gave you complete balance for the last ten years now makes you tired, sore, and leaves you with increased weight. In this cycle, the body becomes catabolic and starts to break down.

My Personal Cycle Three

When I turned thirty-five years of age, I had to change my diet and training philosophy. I was experiencing sore joints and realized I couldn't train like I did in my twenties. By the time I reached forty years of age, I didn't have trouble with my lifestyle. While all my friends were complaining about their health, I felt like a kid. When I reached forty-five years of age, everything started to change. I keep detailed records of my measurements, diet, and exercise programs; any changes I make, I monitor closely to see the effect. I was following the same overall regimen I had used for the last few years, but I noticed I was starting to have trouble sleeping and I was very tired around 3:00 p.m. during the day. The other thing that changed was I noticed my pants getting tighter in the waist. Nothing had changed in my lifestyle program, but my body was falling apart.

I immediately took action and ran some tests on myself. First, I ran some blood tests to make sure that nothing was physiologically wrong. Then I did my body composition to check my muscle-to-fat ratio, and finally, I ran a cardio metabolic stress test (bio-energy test) to make sure my body was producing energy properly and I was exercising in the right heart rate zones. The results were as follows:

1. Blood tests. The tests showed that I was having trouble with my thyroid. This definitely could be the reason for my increased fatigue and enlarged waist size.
2. Body composition. My weight was exactly the same as my last test, but my muscle-to-fat ratio had dropped. This meant I had less muscle and more body fat, again resulting in an increased waist and decreased energy.
3. Cardio metabolic stress test. The results of this test showed me several factors that had changed. First, a decrease in my resting metabolism rate (RMR), which meant my body was burning less calories at rest. Second, my fat burning rate (FBR) and my anaerobic threshold rate (ATR) had changed, and I was exercising too hard causing my body to break down, again resulting in an increased waist and decreased energy.

When I made the adjustments in my program, the results were startling. I dropped my body fat to 10 percent and my waist to thirty-two inches and my energy levels were incredibly high. The adjustments were easy for me. What is remarkable is how much my body changed even though I was already taking extremely good care of it. The changes that happened to me take place in all of us as we enter the third cycle of health.

In the third cycle of health, our hormones will begin to change. Hormones will change in men as much as they will in women; most men have no idea this is happening. When we hear the word *hormones,* we automatically think of sex hormones. These are only one set of hormones. There are metabolic hormones, stress hormones, and regulatory hormones. There are also hormones released from our fat cells, stomach, white blood cells, and more being discovered every day. Here's a quick outline (both women and men):

1. Sex Hormones. The most important ones are testosterone, estrogen, and progesterone. When these hormones are out of balance, no amount of exercise and nutrition is going to work. When our sex hormones are low, we lose muscle, which is the key biomarker of aging, metabolism, and overall health. I will go into more detail later on in the book on how we can naturally rebalance our bodies and when we should consult a doctor. I have found that most men who suffer from low levels of sex hormones reach these low blood serum levels mainly due to a poor lifestyle rather than physiological

reasons and that these levels can be improved with the right diet, exercise, and supplement program.

2. Stress Hormones. When I get to the BioFit cell later in this book, I will go into detail on how the stress hormones react in our body to create our stress response. This is important to understand because if we do not manage these hormones, we cannot possibly manage our health. In the way today's society is built, *I believe stress is the number one cause of breakdown in our health, especially as we age.* The main hormones I focus on here are cortisol, adrenaline, and insulin (which is also a metabolic hormone). There are many other hormones involved such as norephinephrine, epinephrine, dehydroepiandrosterone (DHEA), and many others. I will go into detail on their effects on stress and weight loss later on in the book.

3. Metabolic Hormones. These include the thyroid hormones. I believe in checking the thyroid function in all the cycles of health, but especially in cycle three. If the thyroid isn't functioning at optimal levels, it leads to a cascade of problems—weight gain, fatigue, anxiety, depression, even increases in cholesterol. Other important metabolic hormones include insulin, glucagon, and growth hormone.

4. Regulatory Hormones. These include melatonin, parathyroid hormone, and others. Melatonin is a key hormone we must keep balanced as we age. It sets your twenty-four-hour cycle and is used to make serotonin. If these hormones are out of balance, your moods, sleep, and overall health will suffer.

As you can see, there are many hormones that can get out of balance. This is when your car oil light will come on and it's time to take that car to a service station. It's the same for our body. We need to do a full workup to make sure our bodies are balanced. This is a full physical evaluation including hormones for both men and woman (See appendix B for suggestions). In cycle three, the body can get out of balance and start changing the way it produces energy. As you can see in diagram 3, in the third cycle, the body will start producing anaerobic energy and become catabolic, accelerating the breakdown of the biomarkers of aging.

The stress-response diet will give you what you need to keep the body working at optimal levels for a lifetime. In cycle three, we have to be much more consistent with our diet and exercise. We need to eat the proper combination of food, have the right supplementation, and maintain a healthy schedule to meet the demands of our daily life. At the BioFit Centers, around 30 percent of our clients fall into this cycle.

Cycle Four
Fifty-five Years of Age and Over

At the BioFit Center, our main client base is fifty-five years old and older. Over 30 percent of the clients I see fall into this cycle. Approximately 11 percent of our clients are between sixty to seventy years of age, and 4 percent are over seventy years of age. I was one of the first fitness professionals in the United States to work with these individuals. I designed this program for the cycle four population known as active adults to fit into their active adult communities. The results were amazing.

I currently have clients in their eighties and nineties, enjoying a healthier and pain-free life, thanks to the benefits of the stress-response diet. Overall, as the baby boomers enter the cycle four active adult category, their health and quality of life worsens. The reason behind this situation is simply the lack of an appropriate health and fitness program designed for their specific needs as an active adult. In cycle four, it's not as simple as diet and exercise; the active adult guidelines are very specific for their special needs.

No More Medications
Lilia's Story

Lilia is a seventy-seven-year-old retired nurse who came to see me in search of some answers concerning her exercise and nutrition program. Lilia had been exercising for the last ten years and tried several different diet plans, trying to lose weight. At age fifty-eight, she was diagnosed with high blood pressure and had been on several medications over the years to control it. Lilia had struggled with her weight all her life and she weighed 215 pounds at the height of five feet five inches. Lilia was very proactive when it came to her health and wellness. The diet she followed was a one-thousand-calorie diet, and she was exercising one to two hours daily, mainly doing cardio classes at the local gym.

The first thing I focused on with Lilia was her mind. I had to get her away from that diet, "no pain, no gain" mentality. I taught her how to refocus her goals and her thoughts to help her get the true results that she was seeking. Instead of weight loss, we focused on decreasing size and overall health and increased energy. The second item was to run a series of tests, including laboratory tests with her doctor and the BioFit cardio metabolic stress test. The results gave me the answers I needed to create Lilia's stress-response diet and lifestyle program.

Lilia's laboratory tests revealed that she was having trouble with her thyroid conversion. This meant that her body was producing adequate thyroid-stimulating hormone (TSH) and adequate amounts of thyroxine (T_4), but low amounts of triiodothyronine (T_3). T_4 is 80 percent of the thyroid glands production, but it's the inactive hormone. T_3 is the active hormone; it's five times more active than T_4. For Lilia, her free T_3 was very low. Lilia's doctor did prescribe for her some natural thyroid supplements to strengthen her thyroid response.

Lilia's BioFit cardio metabolic stress test gave me the final answers that I needed to polish her program. The first thing was her combination of foods. She ate a lot of fruit all day long, thinking this is healthy eating; but Lilia's body was having trouble processing carbohydrates. The fruit she was consuming was stopping her body from burning fat. I gave her fruit early in the day along with the proper combinations of food to give her all the nutrients she needed and still manage her insulin response. The second thing the bio-energy test revealed was that she was exercising way out of her aerobic zones. I had to get her to balance her exercise with resistance training and to slow down on the cardio.

Within the first thirty days, Lilia dropped ten pounds and her energy levels began to soar. After six months, she had lost a total of thirty pounds. Finally, after a year following her stress response lifestyle program, she had lost fifty pounds on the scale, gained ten pounds of muscle, and most importantly, she no longer needed medication for her blood pressure. At age seventy-eight, Lilia was biologically thirty. This means she was producing energy like a thirty-year-old. To this day, she is the record holder for biological age versus chronological age.

In cycle four, the key is lifestyle design. I have found that if you exercise too hard or eat the wrong combinations of food, it's virtually impossible to get results. People in cycle four produce the majority of their energy anaerobically, and no diet can work without reversing the energy production back to aerobic. The stress-response diet is designed to repair the metabolism no matter what age you are. With Lilia, it was reversing the way her body was producing energy. That took balancing her thyroid, getting on the proper eating schedule and combinations, and exercising to enhance the body's energy production. Sounds complicated, but it's really easy as you will learn in part 4, "Creating your Lifestyle Program."

Final Notes on the Cycles of Health

1. Many of you might be asking, "What about cycle five?" What I have discovered over the years is that after age fifty-five, the body doesn't change all that much. This means that if you balance your body out at age fifty-five, you will have the same lifestyle program at sixty-five, seventy-five, and eighty-five and beyond, as long as you keep up with the program and do a yearly bio-energy and blood test checkup.

2. It's also important to understand that your chronological age doesn't always determine your cycle of health. If you're thirty years old and your body works like it's fifty-five years of age, I have to treat you like a fifty-five-year-old until I get you balanced out. It's all about how your body is producing energy. *Energy production is the key to health, longevity, and weight loss.*

3. The mind plays a role when it comes to the cycles of health because of the social programming of aging. We are programmed to age a certain way according to the rules of society—age forty, we start to get tired; age fifty, we start medication; age sixty-five, we retire; and so on. As a proud baby boomer, I can tell you the rules are about to change. It's important to never act your age, stay active no matter what, and for God's sake, never retire, there's always something to do. *Keep in mind that the subconscious mind doesn't age.*

4. Remember, you cannot force the body to change. What works in one cycle will not work in another. This doesn't mean that we can't enjoy sports or hard training. It means you have to make sure your body can handle and recuperate from stress by managing the stress response. The stress of family, career, exercise, and today's fast-paced technology world. In the chapter "The Stress-Response Diet," I will give you the tools to recuperate.

Chapter Five

Understanding The Ten Biomarkers of aging and how you can control them

"Age is an issue of mind over matter. If you don't mind, it doesn't matter."

—*Mark Twain*

We learned that as we change cycles of health, our bodies will change the way they physically handle their current lifestyle, even if that lifestyle is healthy. This has to do with the way our bodies produce energy; when this changes, our biomarkers begin to break down. The ten biomarkers are the key for me when I design a personalized nutrition, exercise, and supplement program for a client, and especially when I am monitoring a client's results. The biomarkers will tell me if I have the client on the right regimen. The biomarkers can tell me if I have the proper food combinations, if the client is taking their proper snacks, and if the exercise program is effective. Once I have the client in the right program, I can tell if they are balanced or if I need to change something just by reviewing the individual's markers.

The ten Biomarkers were first established through the research performed by Dr. William Evans. Since the early 1990s, I have used Dr. Evans's research to accurately create tailored lifestyle programs that get remarkable results for my clients.

The biomarkers are so important when assessing the health of an individual, especially as we age. Scientific advancements have enabled many to live longer, but not necessarily healthier lives. Heart disease, cancer, obesity, diabetes, osteoporosis, and serious age-related mental decline such as Alzheimer's are serious problems that could hit epidemic proportions as the baby boomers continue to age. We also have to look at the deterioration of the health of our youth. Only five years ago, I rarely saw children at the BioFit Centers. Today, I have many, even as young as eight years of age. What is surprising is their blood tests results. Every day, I see kids with elevated cholesterol, blood sugar, and broken-down biomarkers.

Another issue that represents a challenge in our world today is the cost of health care. With people living longer lives, but at the same time presenting more age-related health problems, the cost of health care for the general population is affected. In the United States, health care costs jumped to $1.424 trillion in the year 2001, up from $1.310 trillion in the year 2000. Health care spending averages $4,637 per person.

The bottom line is that the world population and their habits have changed drastically in the last twenty years. People are becoming more proactive when it comes to their health and are beginning to seek answers. For people to become truly healthy, they must learn to live healthier lifestyles. New alternatives must be explored. On one hand the diet industry only offers quick and temporary solutions and on the other the medical community is in its infancy in preventive care. The diet industry generates products that make approximately $35 billion in revenue per year by "helping us to lose weight," when in fact the truth is that all we are losing is money.

In the United States, we eat less fat, diet more than any country in the world, and have a fitness club or gym on every other corner. Yet approximately three hundred thousand Americans die every year from obesity-related issues.

As a fellow baby boomer, we have struggled in the era of diet and exercise and are learning that *diets alone don't work*. Not only do they not work, they can potentially affect a person's metabolism and the body's ability to process foods. The truth is we are beginning to discover that it takes a lifestyle change in order to lose weight and keep it off. Dr. Evans's ten biomarkers give you a precise guideline to follow in order to create a true wellness program.

The Biomarkers

Back in the early 1990s, Dr. Evans and Dr. Rosenberg presented evidence that the body's decline is due not to the passing of years, but to the combined effects of inactivity, poor nutrition, and illness. This breakthrough study was what I used to create the stress-response diet. They identified ten biomarkers, the key physiological factors associated with prolonged youth, vitality, health, and metabolism. These ten biomarkers are:

1. muscle mass
2. strength
3. basal metabolic rate
4. body fat
5. aerobic capacity
6. blood pressure
7. blood sugar tolerance
8. cholesterol
9. bone density
10. body temperature regulation

Biomarker One: Muscle Mass

Muscle is the key and the answer to the mysteries of losing weight, becoming healthy, preventing and reversing disease and preserving your lean body mass (muscle). Your body's muscle mass will determine whether or not your cells produce energy properly; in other words, if you're healthy. Your muscle will determine whether your body's aging process is accelerating or slowing down. Your muscle mass will also determine whether you have a strong or a weak metabolism.

You burn approximately 90 percent of your calories within your lean body mass. Our muscle is literally our body's furnace. In order to keep our body young, healthy, and to maintain a strong metabolism, we have to strive to maintain our muscle. In the BioFit cell, we will discuss in detail the true key to turning up your metabolism and increasing health, the *mitochondria*. The mitochondria are the parts of your cells that combine the calories you consume with oxygen and turn this combination into energy, used to run every process in your body. The mitochondria are what dictate the way the body produces energy. When we experience mitochondria decay, our energy production will change. The bottom line is this: more muscle equals more mitochondria. Less muscle, the less mitochondria—this results in less energy.

The challenge is this: it is estimated that at age twenty, we will begin to lose half a pound of muscle every year. Dr. Evans called this sarcopenia (*sarco* meaning "muscle" and *penia* meaning "loss"). At age twenty, the last thing we are thinking about is aging and the breakdown of our body. Sarcopenia is the catabolic breakdown of the body due to aging. Although it's preventable and reversible, most people are unaware of this process. The first time most of us will notice the effects of sarcopenia is usually between the ages of thirty-five and forty years when we enter the second cycle of health. In the third cycle of health, after age forty-five, sarcopenia will begin to accelerate because of hormone changes.

The other challenge we have with sarcopenia and the breakdown of our body is that there are lifestyle factors that can accelerate our breakdown and aging. I have found that these four factors can increase sarcopenia:

1. Stress response. I believe stress is the number one cause of accelerated breakdown and aging of the body. In the BioFit cell, I will go into detail on how stress affects every aspect of our health. For now, it's important to understand that stress is really about balancing three hormones—*cortisol, adrenaline, and insulin.* I have been measuring clients for over twenty-five years with blood tests, body compositions, and the biomarkers. I am truly amazed at the accelerated breakdown of the body at a very young age. I have thirty-year-old clients already showing signs of heart disease and metabolic syndrome (early diabetes). I contribute this to the amount of daily stress and inability to balance the stress response because of the sheer pace of life. Stress management is about keeping the stress response and these hormones balanced so our body can recuperate each day. The stress hormones can cause an imbalance of other hormones in the body, including thyroid.

2. Yo-yo dieting. The fact is, most people's misguided efforts at dieting and exercise will actually promote muscle loss. Every time we lose and regain weight, we will lose muscle. The loss of muscle will decrease our mitochondria and that will bring down our metabolism and accelerate the aging process.

3. Bad habits. Our daily habits will always have an effect on our muscle mass. Smoking, excessive drinking, and the use of all types of drugs will create a breakdown in the muscle. Another bad habit is excessive exercise. After age forty-five, too much exercise is actually worse than not exercising at all.

4. Illness. Anything that limits us from moving will cause an acceleration of muscle breakdown, such as being bedridden. Also, treatments such as chemotherapy and radiation cause extreme sarcopenia. The fact

is every time we get sick, the body will break itself down as part of its survival mechanism.

Biomarker Two: Strength

When I talk about strength, I'm not just talking about how much a person can lift; that's only part of it. I'm talking about how the body is supported. For many years in the United States, most of my clients were 70 years old. Even today, I have probably ninety clients between the ages of seventy and ninety-two years of age. When these clients walk into the BioFit Centers, they have a very distinctive walk. They will be slightly bent over with their bodies leaning forward shaped like a C. These clients always tell me about how they are "shrinking" and, almost always, they complain of joint pain.

The complaints these groups of clients regularly have—of sore joints, weakness, and shrinking—have little to do with their age. The source of the problem is the breakdown of their biomarkers. Our muscles' job is to give support to our skeletal structure. A breakdown in the biomarkers, resulting in less muscle, will cause a chain reaction. The head on our body is heavy. When we lose support, our posture will be affected. This will cause tightening of muscles in the upper back and neck area as the muscles attempt to support the body structure. When this breakdown occurs, our posture will then slump forward.

When there is a breakdown of this biomarker, there will be three vulnerable areas in the body.

1. Knees. The muscles above the knee work like shock absorbers to protect the joint. If we have diminished muscle, there will be no protection for the joint. This means every time we sit, walk, or climb, the joint will take the brunt of the movement instead of the muscle.
2. Lower back/hips. This is a weak link in our body. Without proper muscle support, the lower back and the hips will become vulnerable to injury. When the biomarkers are broken down, the back can get so bad that we can't even sit or stand for prolonged periods.
3. Neck/shoulder area (upper back). When the biomarkers brake down, one of the most vulnerable areas is the neck and upper back. Many elderly people start to develop kyphosis, which appears as a slight

curvature in the upper back, right under the neck. This will form a hump between the head and the upper back.

When it comes to functional fitness such as getting out of a chair, walking up the stairs, or picking up a heavy object, it all has to do with how much muscle mass you have. The muscles are made up of two kinds of fibers—the fast twitch and slow twitch. Slow-twitch fibers are necessary for posture and most low intensity movement. The fast-twitch muscle fibers, in contrast, are the kind we mobilize when we strain to lift heavy objects or do high-intensity exercise. If we are experiencing sarcopenia (breakdown), these fast-twitch muscle fibers will decline rapidly, leaving us weaker.

Biomarker Three: Basal Metabolic Rate (BMR)

The basal metabolic rate (BMR), also referred as the resting metabolic rate, is the number of calories your body burns at rest, in other words, it's your metabolism. Our BMR is directly related to the amount of muscle we have, in other words, to the health status of our biomarkers. This has to do with the mitochondria in our cells. The rate at which the mitochondria transforms food and oxygen into energy is what determines your metabolic rate or your BMR. Our BMR is determined by how many mitochondria we have and how well they burn calories. When we have a breakdown of the biomarkers and lose muscle, we will lower our aerobic capacity or have less oxygen, resulting in a low metabolic rate—BMR. (Note: The cardio-metabolic stress test [bio-energy test] at the BioFit Centers can accurately measure the function of the mitochondria, giving us the most accurate data on a client's metabolism.)

Our metabolism is directly related to the health of our biomarkers. We burn approximately 90 percent of our calories in the muscle; the more muscle mass, the faster the metabolism. It has been shown that obese people have poorly operating and fewer mitochondria. I have found that most of the overweight people I see actually have decreased muscle mass or broken down biomarkers, and this would result in fewer and less functioning mitochondria, thus a slow metabolism. The good news is that this is reversible. Increased muscle improves the biomarkers; you will then increase mitochondria numbers and function. This is how I have been able to keep my own weight off; I took control and changed my metabolism.

Biomarker Four: Body Fat

When I work with clients, the first thing I tell them is our *goal at BioFit is not to lose weight!* Our goal is to lose fat. Most clients' response is: "yeah, yeah, I want to lose fat . . ." Think about it. The diet industry measures your progress by how many pound you have lost. The medical field measures a patient's health by how much they weigh on the scale. Neither of these truly matters, the only things that matter are the muscle-to-fat ratio and the body fat percentage. The stress-response diet is about losing fat and inches, and this fat loss is what translates into health. Our health and the health of our cells are directly determined by how much and where we store our fat.

Science has come to the conclusion that the fat cell is now part of the endocrine system because of the hormones that it releases. The fat cell has a hormonal communication network in the body that will allow us to either burn or store fat. The adipose tissue (fat) releases hormones that affect our metabolism, appetite, and overall health. There are two groups of fat cells. The first group is subcutaneous fat cells that store fat beneath our skin. The second group is visceral fat cells; these are located primarily in the abdomen. These are the cells that produce the hormones that affect our metabolism. When we have excess visceral fat we will then have increased inflammation in the body.

When we talk about inflammation, there are two types. First is what Dr. Barry Sears calls *screaming inflammation*, which is the body's reaction to a cut or a scrape; and the body reacts by getting red, swollen, and experience discomfort and pain on the injured site. The second is called *silent inflammation.* Silent inflammation is asymptomatic, that is, it doesn't manifest itself loudly or obviously; it's silent or passive until it's too late. This type of inflammation is the major cause of stroke, heart disease, diabetes, cancer, Alzheimer's disease, and accelerated aging.

Fat loss is the key to controlling our overall and long-term health. If you have healthy biomarkers, you will attain the body you have always wished for, and you will protect your body from inflammation and disease.

Biomarker Five: Aerobic Capacity

The aerobic capacity has to do with how much oxygen your body has. It is tied into your cardiopulmonary system and the body's ability to transport oxygen effectively to all parts of the body. When our biomarkers break down and we have a decrease in muscle, we will experience a decrease in the number of mitochondria as our muscle cells have one of the highest concentrations of mitochondria. A decrease in mitochondria results in a decrease in your BMR (metabolism).

When our oxygen levels drop, the body changes the way it produces energy. Without enough oxygen, the body is unable to burn as much fat for fuel, thus changing our body's energy production to glucose. When this happens, you will experience two distinct things. One, you will get tired especially in the afternoon; your energy will drop significantly. The second thing that happens is that you begin to lose your concentration and start to forget more. In the BioFit cell, we will go into more detail why this happens. For now, understand that decreased aerobic capacity means less oxygen, which means less fat burning and broken-down biomarkers.

Oxygen is the key to balanced health and weight loss. When our body's oxygen is low, nothing in our body will be able to run at full capacity, including the brain. When you have healthy biomarkers your body automatically will have increased aerobic capacity.

Biomarker Six: Blood Pressure

It truly amazes me every time a thirty-, or even a forty-, year-old walks into my office and tells me that they are suffering from hypertension (high blood pressure). Ten years ago, I never saw these problems in such young groups; today, it's almost daily. The causes of hypertension include a hereditary disposition for the problem. But the thirty-year-old clients with high blood pressure aren't usually coming from heredity, usually, it's their lifestyle. Too much sugar and high consumption of bad fats, salt, alcohol and smoking all combined with high stress levels and too little exercise. Hypertension is heavily implicated in strokes and heart attacks, along with a host of other problems in the body.

Most people show a steady increase in blood pressure as they age. I believe this is directly due to the breakdown of the biomarkers. I believe this because when I reverse clients' biomarkers, I reverse their hypertension. I have had many clients get off blood pressure medications or at least have the medication reduced after becoming biologically fit. Most people believe the first line of defense in treating hypertension is cutting salt and fat from the diet. Only 10 percent of the general population is responsive in that their blood pressure responds to the intake of salt. When it comes to fats, there are five different types, two we have to cut out, and three that are essential to our health and any type of weight loss. I have discovered that one of the biggest dietary changes people can make to control hypertension is controlling the insulin response in the body. The stress-response diet will give you the proper guidelines, the right combination of foods, along with the right timing of your meals and the proper order in which to eat a meal to help you to control your blood pressure.

The other vital key to controlling blood pressure is exercise. Without proper exercise as we age, even if we maintain a perfect diet, it's difficult to keep our blood pressure at healthy levels. The reason again has to do with the biomarkers; a breakdown down in the markers means less oxygen and decreased cardiopulmonary fitness. At the BioFit Centers, we monitor the blood pressure carefully on our heart patients. It's incredible that those with high blood pressure will have lower readings for at least an hour after just one hour of exercise. The good news is that you don't have to kill yourself exercising to see this kind of results, walking is better than running.

Biomarker Seven: Blood Sugar Tolerance

Over the twenty-five years I have been working in the health and fitness field, I have researched the human metabolism extensively. I have concluded that the food pyramid some experts use under the notion of promoting healthy eating is wrong. I knew it was wrong from the testing I was doing on clients, but more importantly, I knew it was wrong from a personal standpoint. My problems with my weight were due to the fact that I didn't process carbohydrates properly. The bottom line was that the food pyramid "low-fat diets" actually made me fatter. Many baby boomers hurt their metabolisms during this low-fat-craze era.

The ability for our body to be able to control our blood sugar is called glucose tolerance. When our biomarkers break down, our body will lose the ability to take up and productively use sugar from our bloodstreams. Every carbohydrate we eat turns into sugar; it doesn't matter what the carbohydrate is, it turns into sugar. Once the sugar enters the bloodstream, the pancreas will swing into action by releasing the hormone insulin. Insulin's job is to get the sugar out of the bloodstream and into the cells. Immediately, insulin begins to stimulate the body's muscle cells (biomarker one) to take in and utilize the glucose circulating in the bloodstream. Muscle tissue is programmed to respond to insulin, it's sensitive to insulin. Healthy biomarkers are the key to blood sugar control as muscle is the primary site for glucose (sugar) disposal.

Over these years, I have been fortunate to work with all age groups. When I first started twenty-five years ago, there was a condition called adult-onset diabetes. This simply meant the body couldn't process the sugar properly as we just talked about. This happened in older adults because as they aged, their biomarkers broke down as a result of less muscle mass. This is what's referred to as type 2 diabetes. Type 1 diabetics do not produce enough insulin from the pancreas to be able to remove sugar from the bloodstream; these diabetics need to take insulin to control their sugar. The truth be told, I no longer believe in adult-onset diabetes; it's simply just type 2 diabetes now. The reason is so many young people are now getting this disease due to the lifestyle they live. It no longer has to do with age; it has to do with the health of the biomarkers. If we don't change, I believe this will become a worldwide epidemic. I say this because of the sheer number of kids I see already beginning to test positive for sugar intolerance.

Metabolic Syndrome

Before leaving "Biomarker Seven: Blood Sugar Intolerance," I want to mention a new syndrome that has developed as a result of blood sugar intolerance called metabolic syndrome. I believe this syndrome is a direct reflection of the diets that were being prescribed in the eighties and nineties. Following the experts' advice, we were following the low-fat food pyramid, low-calorie diets. There was a flood of low-fat foods that hit the market—everything from cookies, crackers, and cereals to ice creams. Since the conception of the high-carbohydrate, low-fat diet approaches, there are twenty million more obese people today. The average American is ten pounds heavier today than he was only five years ago, and when it comes to our children, the situation is even worse.

Many doctors still prescribe these low-fat, high-carbohydrate diets to patients with high cholesterol, high blood pressure, and heart disease. Yet these diets will give the patient constant problems in trying to regulate their sugar levels. I see this happening every day with my clients; they follow their prescribed diet only to develop a new disease, diabetes.

After years of testing clients, I can tell you that these diets do not reduce high blood pressure because they do not promote long-term fat loss. They do not lower cholesterol levels in some cases; they can even increase them. Finally, these diets biggest promotional claim is that you will lose weight, meaning any weight (water or muscle, but most likely not fat).

After so many years of eating the wrong type of carbohydrates and the wrong combinations of food, we have created a new syndrome called *metabolic syndrome X*.

This syndrome is hyperinsulinemia, an identifiable metabolic disorder that makes it impossible to lose weight (fat). This is considered the step before diabetes, but holds implications on its own. First, when you have this syndrome, your sugar levels will fluctuate from one extreme to the other. This causes severe fatigue and loss of concentration. The second symptom is where you store fat when you have this syndrome. Fat storage tends to be around the middle, increasing visceral fat. This causes a cascade of problems from hormone communications to increased inflammation. The great news about metabolic syndrome X is that it's completely reversible, and the stress response diet will give you all the tools you need to turn this around in just a few weeks. The key is following the right program for your body as we will discuss in part 4, "Creating your Lifestyle Program."

Biomarker Eight: Cholesterol

When I review a client's blood test results I look at how their body is reacting to his/her diet, exercise and supplement regimen. I am not looking for anything wrong; These interpretations allow me to really tailor the clients' program to fit the way their metabolism and bodies are working. If the client's labs are off, I immediately send them to their doctor. I can tell you that blood tests can tell us so much more than whether we are just sick or not. In appendix B, I have included a list of labs for the different cycles of health and what I look at when putting together a clients' program.

Cholesterol is a fatty substance that's a necessary component for the health of our body. It plays an essential role in the construction of cell membranes and is essential for our sex hormones to stay balanced. It circulates in the bloodstream in association with protein, in combined entities known as *lipoproteins*. I always tell my clients that I am not concerned with their total cholesterol number. I am concerned with the breakdown of the lipoproteins; this determines if you have good or bad cholesterol. Here is how the cholesterol breaks down into your lipid panel:

1. Low-density lipoprotein (LDL). This is the dreaded "bad cholesterol" that can collect and form deposits in our arteries, which is called atherosclerosis. Imagine your arteries are like a pipe and LDL cholesterol

is the sludge that blocks the flow of the water in the pipe. LDL cholesterol rise for several reasons:

- You are consuming too many saturated or trans fats in your diet. These are whole dairy, butter, fatty meats, along with the dreaded potato chips, crackers, and overall junk food.
- Your body isn't processing sugar efficiently (biomarker seven). Eating processed/high-glycemic carbohydrates like white bread, pastries, candies, and sugary drinks, along with most junk food, will play a major role in raising the bad cholesterol.
- This can be from changes in the hormones in the body, especially changes in the thyroid can cause cholesterol to rise. Genetics also play a strong role in the rise of LDL cholesterol. The BioFit phase one menu is especially designed to help lower cholesterol levels. I have seen clients drop one hundred points in as little as thirty days. I have found if your cholesterol is high genetically, diet and exercise alone will not be able to lower it.

2. High-density lipoprotein (HDL). HDL cholesterol is referred to as the "good cholesterol." HDL cholesterol removes the excess cholesterol lining from our blood vessels, then brining it back to the liver for reprocessing. This keeps our arteries clear and can decrease our risk of heart attack and stroke.

It is essential to our long-term health and disease prevention to raise our good HDL cholesterol. For every one point increase in HDL, there is a 3 percent decrease in a person's risk of suffering a fatal heart attack. The stress-response diet is designed with a special menu and exercise plan to help you increase your good cholesterol. Here are a few lifestyle changes that will positively affect your HDL:

- Exercise. This is a major key into raising our good cholesterol.
- Quit smoking. This can raise the HDL cholesterol immediately.
- Decrease your body fat: This has to do with the proper combinations of food. We will discuss this further in chapter 4, "Creating your Lifestyle Program."
- Eat good fats. The essential fatty acids must be balanced in your diet to increase the HDL cholesterol.

- Add fiber. Fiber found in foods such as fruits, vegetables, nuts, certain grains can boost your HDL.

There are also medications like certain statins and niacin that can help balance your HDL/LDL ratios.

3. Triglycerides. Triglyceride levels are often overlooked but are a key element I use when preparing a menu for a client. Triglycerides aren't usually given the importance that cholesterol levels are given, but they are an important factor in assessing the destructive process of atherosclerosis and heart disease. Over the years, I have worked with many doctors and I have found that their attention is usually focused on the cholesterol levels, and not the triglycerides. This is changing quickly as there is more and more evidence between the connection of elevated triglycerides and cardiovascular disease and diabetes.

Triglycerides are important fats that fuel our organ function, except for the brain, which runs on glucose. It's when our triglycerides are elevated that we get into trouble. When they are elevated, usually the weight will be around our middle. As we discussed in biomarker four, this is the weight that will promote inflammation in our body. The main cause of elevated triglycerides is that our body is not processing carbohydrates properly. This can come from physiological changes in the body or the consumption of the wrong types of carbohydrates, even the timing of when you consume carbohydrates, and the amount of fiber in your diet has an effect on triglycerides.

The Overlooked triglycerides

As I mentioned, triglycerides are often overlooked when the doctor is assessing our cholesterol. In fact, a client with elevated triglycerides generally will have LDL cholesterol (bad) lower than normal. This is very deceiving because when triglycerides are elevated, another type of cholesterol will raise VLDL cholesterol (very low-density lipoproteins), which I will discuss next.

The bottom line is elevated triglycerides are associated with premature coronary heart disease in people with special types of diseases such as diabetes, severe high cholesterol levels, fatty liver, and chronic kidney disease. Lab reference ranges state that triglycerides should be below 150 mg/dl. I believe that they should always be below 100 mg/dl for optimal fat burning and inflammation control. In most cases, I find that clients on the stress response diet can drop triglyceride levels within the first thirty days.

4. Very low-density lipoprotein (VLDL). As I mentioned earlier, when triglycerides are elevated, so will the VLDL cholesterol. "VLDL are large lipoproteins rich in triglycerides. VLDL circulates through the blood giving up their triglycerides to fat and muscle tissue until the VLDL remnants are modified and converted into LDL" (www.audioenglish. net. Dictionary entry overview.) This is why when a client has elevated triglycerides, they will usually have low LDL. This is deceiving because the VLDL will be elevated, and it has to be considered bad cholesterol, in fact, very bad cholesterol. When working with a client with elevated triglycerides, I will add LDL and VLDL levels together to get a more accurate assessment of their lipid panel.

In conclusion, the total cholesterol/HDL is important to our overall health; but the balance of our overall lipid panel is the key to being bio-fit. When our biomarkers are broken down, our body's lipids will become unbalanced. As our biomarkers become healthy, our lipids will balance, allowing us to control lifestyle related conditions such as heart disease, diabetes, and even aging (inflammation).

Biomarker Nine: Bone Density

Our bones lose calcium as we age. Bone density also deteriorates when we lose muscle mass (biomarker breakdown). Loss of muscle mass makes the skeletal structure weaker, less dense, and more brittle. If this breakdown goes too far, the person will develop osteoporosis. Our bone density is protected by proper nutrition balance, weight-bearing exercise, and the right supplements—all which will be discussed in part 4, "Creating your Lifestyle Program."

Biomarker Ten: Body Temperature Regulation

This marker usually presents itself in my older clients, seventy years and above. One of the challenges I have with these clients is to get them to drink enough water during the day to keep the body hydrated. As we age, our thirst mechanism begins to shut down; we don't get thirsty. Yet our fluid output stays the same or even increases. The end result is dehydration. This will cause the body to have trouble maintaining an internal temperature of 98.6 degrees Fahrenheit, making an elderly person vulnerable to hot and cold weather.

These ten biomarkers are the key to properly access a person's health. When we have decreased biomarkers, there will be a domino effect—one marker leads to the next.

Chapter Six

Biomarkers: The Domino Effect

"Everything in nature is a cause from which there flows some effect."
—Spinoza

The lifestyle we live on a consistent and daily basis will determine whether we are catabolic (breaking down-aging) or anabolic (balanced-recuperating). Modern culture and its fast-paced approach places an enormous amount of stress on each individual. Experts believe that our bodies break down and age more rapidly because of this stress. They also believe that much of the increase in lifestyle related illness such as heart disease and diabetes can also be linked directly or indirectly to stress.

I have to strongly agree with these experts. Stress is a key factor in causing accelerated aging and decreased health. The challenge we face is that we cannot get rid of stress; we can only manage it. Our stress response is part of our survival DNA; we cannot simply shut it off. It is necessary, in order to lose weight and create optimal health, that we learn how to manage stress. The stress-response diet will offer you all the tools needed to create the lifestyle you need to easily take control of the stress response in your life.

The key biomarker is biomarker one (muscle). If this marker is breaking down, it will cause what I call a domino effect with the other nine markers. Stress, as we mentioned in biomarker one, is the major cause of accelerated muscle breakdown and the collapse of the biomarkers. When our daily stress goes unmanaged and we become catabolic, our biomarkers will begin to breakdown. Let's take a look at this effect and how it relates to your body's health, metabolism and aging.

1. Muscle. Our muscle breaks down due to stress and an unbalanced lifestyle. This breakdown begins to create a domino effect leading to the next marker.
2. Strength. With the declining muscle, comes less strength. Our posture begins to change. We develop back, neck, and knee problems along with body aches and joint pain. Because of this discomfort, we cannot exercise and start becoming more sedentary, which accelerates the breakdown of the biomarkers.
3. Basal metabolic rate (BMR). Our bodies burn approximately ninety percent of its calories in the muscle; it's the body's furnace. Our bodies begin to burn less calories even when we sleep. We begin to feel sluggish as our body no longer produces energy properly. Our energy levels are low, we begin to get cravings for sweets, and develop mood swings.
4. Body fat. Our clothes are now beginning to get tight, and our weight starts to climb. We begin to gain weight especially in the middle, around our belly and buttocks. We begin to feel frustrated and, in some cases, depressed due to our uncontrollable weight gain. At this point, diets no longer are effective.

Note:

The first four biomarkers are the cosmetic markers; they determine what your body looks like. I usually see people in their late twenties and early thirties beginning to show problems with the first four markers (in recent years, I have seen more and more teenagers with signs of breakdown in these four markers). This is like a warning message the body sends. These people do not feel bad yet; the main reason they come to see me is because they are having trouble losing weight. Their main focus is always lowering their weight on the scale. What they fail to understand is that a breakdown of the first four biomarkers is what leads to the breakdown of the next four, and that's when our health begins to break down. If you are showing signs of deficiency in the first four markers (muscle, strength, BMR, and body fat), this leads to problems with the next four markers (aerobic capacity, blood pressure, blood sugar intolerance, and cholesterol profile).

When the biomarkers break down, the way you look will start to change; but more importantly, what happens inside of your body is what truly will affect your health. Muscle is a metabolically active tissue; one pound of muscle burns approximately ten calories. Fat is metabolically inactive, it doesn't burn any calories. If your body composition changes, your active tissue drops (muscle), and your inactive tissue (fat) rises, your body composition changes for the worse and you begin to look overweight. As the side effect of this equation, your body chemistry begins to change for the negative. Once people reach this stage of biomarker breakdown, they then begin to develop conditions and symptoms related to the next four biomarkers. This usually happens during the second cycle of health.

Let's continue to see what happens to the biomarkers as the result of the breakdown of the first four. The domino effect carries on:

5. **Aerobic capacity.** Aerobic capacity is not the same as cardiovascular fitness. Aerobic capacity is how much oxygen is in your body. When our bodies have decreased oxygen, two distinct things will begin to take place. First, your energy levels will begin to drop (especially in the afternoon). Second, you will begin to forget things and have trouble concentrating. This biomarker is the key for longevity, fat loss, and overall health and performance.

6. **Blood pressure.** Hypertension (elevated blood pressure) is a devastating condition that rarely shows any symptoms until it's too late. When our body's oxygen drops, our blood pressure will begin to rise. Working with doctors in Panama City, Panama, I found it amazing that patients that came to Panama from Colombia would sometimes have to cut their medication by half just from the changes in altitude. This is due to their oxygen levels changing. At the BioFit Centers, we monitor the client's blood pressure closely. We have found that when a person becomes biologically fit, their blood pressure will balance out and decrease if it was high prior to becoming "healthier." For those clients on medications, this means a reduction on their dosages (many clients of all ages get off blood pressure medications).

7. **Blood sugar tolerance.** When the biomarkers are broken down, one of the key links in the domino effect is the body's ability to process carbohydrates. Our blood sugar tolerance reflects how our body controls its blood sugar levels. As we get older, we will start having problems processing carbohydrates in our diet. This means that a balanced diet that worked in one cycle of health may not work in the next cycle. This is directly due to biomarker breakdown. This breakdown is what leads to what is called adult-onset diabetes

(type 2). In modern times, there has been an increase of type 2 diabetes due to higher levels of stress and a more sedentary lifestyles, especially in young people. When we start having trouble processing carbohydrates, the chemistry of the diet is more important than the calories.

8. **Cholesterol.** As your biomarkers deteriorate, your body will start to produce more cholesterol. Elevated cholesterol is beginning to reach epidemic proportions as more and more young people are being diagnosed with this condition. As the biomarkers break down the body will begin to have trouble processing carbohydrates and this will begin to cause a rise in cholesterol. There are certain diseases that can cause elevation in cholesterol levels such as thyroid disease, certain kidney diseases, diabetes, and liver disease such as a fatty liver.

9. **Bone density.** When all the biomarkers weaken, so does your ability to maintain your body's bone density. This happens from the lack of muscle mass, which leads to the lack of energy, which leads to a sedentary lifestyle. Other factors are the body's changing nutritional needs and hormone changes as our bodies age and break down. If you are losing bone density, you are definitely losing lean body mass and accelerating the aging process.

10. **Body temperature regulation.** For many years, I worked with an active adult population where the average age was seventy years old. I noticed that most of the older people I worked with had trouble regulating their body's temperature. They may be in a warm climate and feel cold or vice versa. The reason for this stems from their inability to get thirsty regularly. This lack of thirst means less water consumption, even though their output remains the same. All of this leads to a state of dehydration. This is a quote of an excerpt from Dr. Deepak Chopra's book, *Ageless Body, Timeless Mind*, "Not drinking enough water everyday is one of the most common conditions in old age, chronic dehydration being a major cause of preventable aging. It is an avoidable complication that leads to many problems."

You can see how the domino effect from the breakdown of the ten biomarkers accelerates aging and disease. The stress-response diet gives you all the tools to prevent and reverse the domino effect at any age or any physical shape you are currently in.

The Ten Biomarkers of Aging:
Reversing the Domino Effect

Joe is a seventy-four-year-old patient of one of the cardiologists that we work closely with. Joe had undergone a triple bypass a few years back, and it seemed that he was going to need a pacemaker. Joe's cardiologist wanted us to help him lose some body fat in a sensible manner. When Joe first started the program, he couldn't walk for more than five minutes at a time and was very weak in all his functional exercises. Slowly, by practicing our resistance training and nutritional guidelines, Joe began to reverse his biomarkers. He began to gain strength quickly,—along with his energy levels which were on the rise.

Joe was able to lose twenty-six pounds on the scale and gained ten pounds of muscle. This means that he actually lost thirty-six pounds of fat. The most important thing is that because of the change in his body composition (biomarkers), his blood pressure medication had to be lowered to fit his new biologically younger body. Imagine the change in Joe's life. When Joe started, he was biologically eighty-five years of age, after as little as six weeks on the program, he tested at sixty years biologically. Joe was experiencing freedom he hadn't had in years, the freedom to be healthy.

It is important to know that once you begin a healthy lifestyle, your biomarkers immediately begin to improve. As you implement the stress-response diet, your body becomes anabolic and uses oxygen and fat for energy and you become biologically younger. Our biological age is determined simply by how our body produces energy. As soon as you start practicing the five bio-links, biomarker one (muscle mass), improves. The average muscle gain for a seventy-year-old client is approximately ten to twelve pounds in about twelve weeks, given that they practice all the bio-links. The quick response in older clients is partly due to what is called muscle memory. Muscle remembers how to work, and it comes back. In fact, people who were athletic in their younger years are able to gain muscle strength faster than those who weren't.

As muscle comes back, so does strength (biomarker two). When you raise your muscle mass and strength, you are also raising your basal metabolic rate (biomarker three). This means your body is now burning more calories, even when you sleep. Then you will notice that your clothes no longer fit tight as now you have less body fat (biomarker four), your clothing becomes loose. At this point, many clients will come to me and say, "I don't get it. My weight hasn't changed much, but I'm down two dress sizes," or "I had to take my belt down three holes. My clothes are falling off me!" Muscle weighs more than fat. When you change your biomarkers, you automatically change your body composition, and this is the key to optimal health.

When you improve your muscle mass, strength, BMR, and lower your body fat, the next thing that will happen to your body is probably the most important change. You begin to improve your aerobic capacity (biomarker four), the amount of oxygen that can travel through your body at a given time. This translates into having to make less effort to move. You feel more aware, and your body feels more agile. Some people report that they simply sleep better and have less trouble focusing or concentrating.

With the increased aerobic capacity, the next biomarker influenced will be your blood pressure. Approximately four out of five clients who come to our center with high blood pressure end up having to lower the dosage of their medication after just a few weeks of following the stress-response diet.

Many people suffer high blood pressure mainly due to a genetic predisposition. These clients may never be able to live without medication, but following the program helps to keep the dosage of medication under control as well as avoiding any potentially related illness attributed to high blood pressure. On the other side of the coin, there are clients with high blood pressure due to bad habits, bad diets, and excessive levels of stress. Two out four of these clients are able to get off medication after only being in the program for a few months. The stress-response diet gives you the specific guidelines to change the variables that result in high blood pressure.

With the total reconstruction of the biomarkers, you can also reverse blood sugar level problems (biomarker seven). You can create more muscle, have less body fat, and increase aerobic capacity. The sum total of these improvements is better-functioning cells. When our cells function well, we produce energy using fat, which allows our sugar levels to stay balanced. This healthy cell function that promotes fat burning will also keep our cholesterol (biomarker eight) under control. Biomarker nine, bone density has a direct relation to healthy muscle mass (biomarker one), which also correlates with body temperature regulation (biomarker ten). Everything fits like a puzzle; all the pieces go together.

Protecting our biomarkers and keeping them healthy is the key to *optimal health and total wellness*. In the next chapter, we will discuss the number one factor that causes biomarker breakdown, the stress response.

Chapter Seven

Creating Biologically Fit Cells

Lack of activity destroys the good condition of every human being, while movement and methodical physical exercise save it and preserve it.

—Plato

I have to say that the life I live is never on the boring side. I travel the world teaching people the wellness culture of becoming and living biologically fit. Last week alone, I met clients from Sweden, Australia, Canada, Costa Rica, and Peru. In my travels, I deal with many high-level professionals, politicians, businessmen, and other people from all walks of life, all of which have elevated levels of stress in their day-to-day lives. The main complaints I hear from these clients is that their stress levels are high, they have low energy levels, and they have trouble sleeping. Many of them have borderline hypertension (high blood pressure), high cholesterol, and are taking several medications for everything from reflux to helping them sleep. Most of these clients were in their thirties, except one that was forty years of age. Every day, I see thirty-year-old clients with hypertension, elevated sugar, and blood pressure problems. They are thirty years of age, but are fifty-five years biologically. Therefore, I have to treat them as if they were fifty-five years old in order to get results. On the other hand, I have seventy-year-old clients who are also biologically fifty-five. It simply doesn't matter how old you are; What matters is how old you are biologically.

For many years, biological age was something we would estimate using the biomarkers. Today, we can actually measure it. Our biological age has to do with the health of our cells and how our body is producing energy. For the last six years, I have used a BioFit cardio metabolic stress test to measure biological stress to test my clients' biological age and other variables. The bio-energy test can accurately access an individual's biological age. The software for this test was developed by Dr. Frank Shallenberger. In his first book entitled *Bursting with Energy*, he proposed a new theory about aging and the breakdown of the body. His theory is referred to as energy deficit disorder, which simply means that as our body's cells begin to produce less and less energy we begin to age. This concept changed the way many scientists view aging. To understand this, let's take a look at how our cells work.

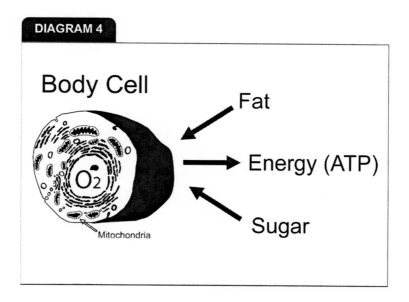

Our body has trillions of cells. These cells have two fuel sources to create energy, fat, and sugar (glucose). These fuels enter the cell, where the cell has many tiny computers called mitochondria. The mitochondria combine the calories we consume with oxygen and then turn this mixture into energy that will be used to run everything in your body. This energy is called adenosine triphosphate (ATP) and is stored in a special molecule until the energy is needed. When our energy levels are high, we have a lot of ATP; when our energy levels are low, we have little ATP. Every single aspect of the functioning of our cells and organs is completely dependent on having an adequate amount of ATP.

When we are young and balanced, we will use fat to create our energy. As we get older (usually starting the second cycle of health), we will start to use more sugar to create our energy and we stop using fat. This change in energy production also occurs when our body gets out of balance. When our body stops using fat as its main fuel source and begins to use mainly sugar, this is when our body will begin to break down. While the cells of our body have two fuel sources, fat and sugar, the cells of our brain only has one fuel source and that is sugar. The brain cells and nervous system uses glucose (sugar) exclusively for energy. The brain has been referred to as a glucose hog, gobbling about sixty-six percent (or two-thirds) of the body's circulating carbohydrates while you are at rest even though the brain weighs less than two pounds.

When our body shifts from fat to glucose (sugar) for its fuel, this is when we will begin to gain weight, have less energy, and start to feel old. Our body can only store a small amount of sugar at a given time. If the body is using sugar for fuel and the brain needs sugar to function, the body will go as far as to break down muscle to produce this sugar. It is estimated that our body can only hold a two- to three-hour supply of sugar. *Our body is very efficient in storing fat and very inefficient at storing sugar.* When our cells suffer this imbalance, you will experience what is commonly known as cravings. Most people have no idea that it doesn't matter if you crave bread, pasta, rice, potato, or if you crave ice cream, chocolate, or cookies; it's all the same craving, it's the commander in chief of the body, the brain, asking for fuel. When I see clients who crave sweets, it's a sure sign that their body is out of balance and breaking down. (See diagram D5, energy production)

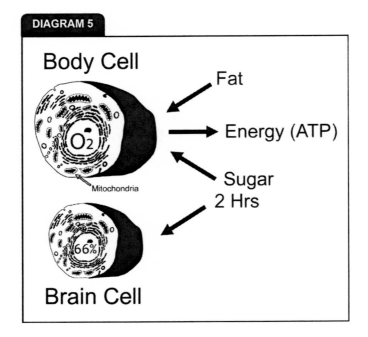

The key for our overall health, energy, proper weight, and age management is making sure our body's cells are balanced and producing energy properly. To have this balance and optimal health, we need to use fat to fuel the cells of our body. When we burn fat for energy, this allows the sugar to be used by the brain, thus creating balance. These are BioFit cells (they are biologically fit).

Fat-Burning Metabolism

One of the elements required for the cells to burn fat is oxygen. If you don't have enough oxygen in your cells, it really doesn't matter how good your diet is, you will not burn fats efficiently. When we are healthy and fit, we will almost exclusively burn fat for energy. As we age or when we get out of balance, our metabolism will shift from primarily burning fat for energy to primarily burning sugar. This fat-to-sugar shift can be directly linked to the breakdown of the ten biomarkers. Here is what happens:

1. The biomarkers break down, starting with a decrease in muscle and an increase in fat, changing your muscle-to-fat ratio.
2. With the change in our muscle-to-fat ratio, our aerobic capacity decreases, lowering the oxygen in our body. This will cause a shift from fat-to-sugar metabolism, causing the body to burn more sugar.
3. Our body can only store small amounts of sugar, thus creating an imbalance of energy production. This results in a continuous depletion of glucose stores (sugar) and unevenness in our overall energy production. To compensate for these roller-coaster energy levels, it forces you to eat more carbohydrates in order to replenish the low sugar. This cycle is what causes cravings for carbohydrates and sweets.
4. The more we crave and eat carbohydrates, the more sugar we put in the body and the more insulin we release. The cells that allow the sugar to get out of the bloodstream become resistant and weak. This will result in increases in blood sugar levels and insulin resistance (the body doesn't process carbohydrates anymore).
5. The body is now continuously on a sugar roller coaster, high and low. We eat more carbohydrates because our body is craving them, giving us a high, only to experience more cravings in a short time period when we hit the low. The body then adapts to this dietary

shift by focusing more and more on burning sugar and less and less on burning fat.

6. The body now cannot process the sugar properly, causing the body to convert the sugar to fat. This will result in an increase in cholesterol and especially triglyceride levels. The weight gain is usually around the middle. This weight will increase inflammation in the body, increasing our risks of heart disease, stroke, diabetes, and Alzheimer's disease.

7. When the body burns less fat, you will have an increase in your body fat percentages. With the increase in body fat, the insulin resistance increases, blocking any attempt for the body to use its fat stores.

8. Finally, as your body's response to the imbalance of a fat-to-sugar shift continues, your body will attempt to balance itself. Cortisol is the body's main stress hormone; it's also the primary hormone your body uses to balance the effects of insulin. The increased levels of insulin causes your adrenal glands to compensate by increasing production and levels of cortisol, causing an imbalance of the stress hormones and increasing the breakdown of the biomarkers.

This breakdown is what used to be called aging. It has been accepted at certain ages that we will lose our eyesight, become fatigued, and develop diabetes and heart disease. It's also accepted that as we age, our libido decreases and we retire. the truth is that none of this has to happen, it doesn't matter what your age is. What truly matters is how old you are biologically. Your *biological age* is determined by how your body is producing energy. In other words, are you producing energy like a thirty-year-old or are you producing energy like a seventy-year-old? Your chronological age doesn't matter!

The BioFit cell is the key to healthy energy production. It's also the key to creating a strong metabolism, permanent weight loss, and preventing lifestyle related diseases. The BioFit Cell will use fat for its resting energy, allowing the sugar to fuel its anaerobic needs as well as the brain. As we talked about in "Biomarker One: Muscle," the key component for a healthy cell is the *mitochondria*.

Mitochondria: Creating a Strong Fat-Burning Metabolism

Jamie is a forty-nine-year-old computer programmer, married, and the father of two children. He had lost fifty pounds of weight two years earlier on a low-fat diet and his own exercise plan. When he came to see me, he was complaining of fatigue, and despite following a strict diet and exercise regimen, he was unable to drop the last twenty-five pounds of weight that he believed he needed to lose. He said that he was exercising about two hours a day, six days a week. He was doing intense cardiovascular exercise that included aerobic and spinning classes, along with running and some kickboxing. Jamie was having trouble sleeping at night and complained of increased memory loss.

Because of Jamie's intense exercise schedule, we ran a BioFit cardio metabolic test. This test measures the amount of oxygen he consumed and the amount of carbon dioxide he exhaled while exercising and at rest. This gave us an indirect measurement of how his metabolism was working. What determines a healthy metabolism is the ability to burn calories proficiently, and this ability is directly linked to the efficiency and number of mitochondria we have in our cells. The mitochondria, along with oxygen, take the food that we eat and burn it to make energy in our bodies.

The amount of oxygen we are able to breathe per minute determines how many calories we burn and the strength of our metabolism. The more oxygen you breathe, the more calories you are able to burn and the more fat you will use for energy. BioFit cardio metabolic stress test takes this information from the exercise and resting metabolism test and tells us what the individual needs in order to increase their metabolism and rebalance their body.

Jamie's test results revealed that for his age, height, weight and gender, he had a low VO_2 max. This meant that he consumed much less oxygen than he should, and this resulted in increased fatigue and a sluggish metabolism. The BioFit cardio metabolic stress test also showed a decrease in his adrenal function, which meant that he was overtraining and increasing the amount of stress in his body. Finally, the test showed that Jamie wasn't processing carbohydrates properly, which meant his current diet was blocking his energy production and decreasing his metabolism.

The first thing we did with Jamie was to establish an exercise program that would increase his metabolism and fat-burning ability. We established his proper heart rate zones according to his test results. We then gave him a specific type of training called interval training. Jamie would reach the high end of his heart rate zone for one minute and then go to his low end for three minutes. He followed that regimen of intervals for thirty minutes, and then he would spend an additional twenty to thirty minutes at his fat burning rate (FBR). This type of training strengthens the mitochondria's ability to use oxygen more efficiently, thus allowing the body's metabolism to increase and burn more fat.

The other vital exercise component for Jamie was to add resistance training twice a week. When we tested his muscle-to-fat ratio, it was 3.3:1—way below the 5:1 ratio for optimal health. This meant that his biomarkers were broken down. By adding in the resistance training, we would improve his ratios, body composition, and his resting metabolism. By increasing the muscle, we increase his aerobic capacity (oxygen) and we increase the number of mitochondria in the muscle cells, turning Jamie's metabolism up full blast.

The second part of Jamie's program was to change his diet. Jamie's test showed clearly that his body was not properly processing carbohydrates, thus blocking his body's ability to burn fat. Finally, we gave him the correct combination of supplements that his body needed to help him balance out and get his metabolism burning.

In less than four months, Jamie's results were incredible. He dropped eighteen pounds on the scale, but also gained six pounds of muscle. His body fat percentage went from 23.5 percent to 18.9 percent, and his muscle-to-fat ratio went from 3.3:1 to 4.2:1. His energy levels were now high and he was sleeping without any trouble.

Special note on the BioFit cardio metabolic stress test:

During my career, I have used the VO_2 max test to establish many of the exercise guidelines that my clients use, but for the last couple of years, I have mainly used the bio-energy test. This test is so much more than a VO_2 max; it's a VO_2 max-plus. It is designed to interpret the results of the cardio-metabolic test in a way that allows us to create a complete and custom made program to rebalance our client's health and metabolism. I have found after, doing hundred of these tests, that the results I get from the bio-energy test match the client's blood tests results. In Jamie's case, his tests showed very low cortisol, which means his stress hormones were out of balance and basically he was overtraining. He had elevated inflammation markers, elevated glucose levels along with increased triglycerides, and low DHEA levels. The bottom line is that the blood tests matched his BioFit cardio metabolic stress test. I find this test an essential tool for anyone who wants to truly create a tailored lifestyle program that gets results.

Boosting Your Metabolism

The mitochondria are the key to whether you have a strong or weak metabolism. A single cell can have two hundred to two thousand or more mitochondria. Your metabolism is established by the rate that your mitochondria transform food and oxygen into energy. The two factors that will determine your metabolism are the efficiency of your mitochondria and the sheer number of mitochondria you have. The cells that contain the greatest numbers of mitochondria are the heart, liver, and your muscle.

Healthy biomarkers are the key to a strong metabolism as muscle is the key to healthy biomarkers. The more muscle you have, the more mitochondria you will have and the faster your metabolism. With the increase of muscle, you increase your aerobic capacity (oxygen), allowing your mitochondria to efficiently burn calories (fat) and oxygen, creating an abundance of energy. Muscle is a key player in creating an optimal metabolism and permanent weight loss. Muscle is metabolically active; it burns around seventy times as many calories as fat. Having the proper muscle-to-fat ratio or healthy biomarkers is the only way you can lose fat and keep it off. When we diet, we lose muscle (I will discuss this in detail in the bio-links), and when we lose muscle, we destroy our metabolism. It's the reason diets can't and don't work.

I never had a strong metabolism while I was growing up; it wasn't until I started to lift weights in my twenties that everything in my life changed. Obese people have fewer and poorly functioning mitochondria than thin people do. To change this and our metabolism, we have to improve our muscle, in turn improving our biomarkers and becoming BioFit. In part 4, "Creating you Lifestyle Program," I will give you the easy-to-use tools to change your metabolism forever.

Mitochondrial Damage

The number of mitochondria that you have is essential for a strong fat-burning metabolism and your overall health. The second part of the equation is the health and functionality of your mitochondria. The mitochondria are very complex structures; their ability to function is influenced by diet, hormone levels, vitamins, minerals, toxicity, and genetics. As we age, our mitochondria become more vulnerable to damage.

When the mitochondria become damaged, this will drastically decrease your energy production, causing you to age much more rapidly and become vulnerable to many types of diseases. This damage is caused by oxidative stress and free radicals. Oxidative stress occurs naturally during the process of turning calories to energy from food and oxygen from air into usable energy for the body.

When the fuel enters the cell, the mitochondria take this fuel and create a fire inside the cell. Think of a campfire. When the fire is burning, you will have sparks fly off the flame; these sparks are representative of free radicals. Free radicals cause the condition of oxidative stress. This process can be seen in our everyday lives. For example, take a bite of an apple and walk away for a few hours; when you return, the apple is brown. It's the same process that causes a car to rust.

When oxidative stress occurs inside our bodies, it causes us to kind of rust on the inside. This causes mitochondrial dysfunction and contributes to increased aging of the body. Free radicals, when out of control due to the lack of antioxidants, trigger a cascade of health problems that include increased inflammation, diabetes, memory loss, and a decreased metabolism resulting in weight gain.

Creating free radicals and oxidative stress is a normal part of our everyday metabolism. What protects our cells and our health is antioxidants. Antioxidants protect you against weight gain, inflammation, and diabetes. They are essential to keeping a healthy fat-burning metabolism and optimal energy levels. It's essential to obtain antioxidants from a healthy diet and proper supplementation, especially as we age. When our cells are balanced, we will use fat for energy. When we get out of balance and switch from a fat-burning to a sugar-burning metabolism, this is when we gain weight and our body ages and breaks down. The key to staying young and energetic at any age is maintaining a healthy fat metabolism from our balanced cells.

Chapter Eight

Burning Fat as Fuel is what truly matters

Those who think they have not time for bodily exercise will sooner or later have to find time for illness.

—Edward Stanley

What Prevents Fat Burning?

Now you know that burning fat for fuel is crucial for our overall health and longevity. I have found over the years of studying with many doctors that there are ten variables that prevent fat burning.

1. insulin resistance
2. hormone deficiencies
3. excessive carbohydrate intake
4. insufficient sleep
5. carnitine deficiency
6. CoQ_{10} deficiency
7. good fats deficiency
8. excessive ingestion of trans fats
9. vitamin-mineral deficiency
10. stress

Ten Reasons Why the Body Stops Burning Fat

1. Insulin Resistance

Insulin is one of the main hormones we must balance if we want to lose weight. It also plays a key role in balancing the stress response, energy levels, and our overall health. Every time we eat carbohydrates, they are broken down into sugar. All carbohydrates become sugar—the good and the bad. The way your body processes carbohydrates will indicate how balanced and healthy you are.

After we eat a meal that contains carbohydrates and the digestive system breaks it down into sugar, the sugar is then absorbed into the bloodstream and immediately carried to the liver for processing. After the liver completes its job of processing it, the sugar is then released into the bloodstream, causing our sugar levels to rise. The rise in sugar causes our pancreas to release the hormone insulin. Insulin's job is to get the sugar out of the bloodstream and into the cells where the body will turn them into energy.

One of the most important factors that determine whether we have a proper fat-burning metabolism is what I call insulin management. Managing our insulin response is key to burning fat and managing energy levels. The combinations and timing of the foods we eat play an essential role in this process. When you consume the wrong combinations of foods, your body will release a hormone that will essentially shut off fat burning. That hormone is insulin.

The Low-Fat Sham

In the 1990s we followed the advice of the "experts" and most of us used the government-sponsored food pyramid. We were all on low-fat diets, faithfully counting every calorie and fat gram, yet we kept getting fatter. Since the conception of the high-carbohydrate/low-fat diet approach over a decade ago, there are millions more obese people today, yet the medical community continues to stand by this dietary approach.

The most recent studies have shown that the high-carbohydrate diet isn't effective for long-term fat loss. What I have discovered over the years is that there are some people who need more carbohydrates than others in their diets. There just isn't one right diet. I have also dicovered that high carbohydrate diets fail more as we age. Once we enter the second cycle of health around thirty-four to thirty-five years of age, our bodies cannot process carbohydrates as efficiently. This is the cycle of health in which the body becomes more insulin resistant. If you consume the wrong carbohydrates or too many carbohydrates, you can become insulin resistant at any age. I have treated twelve- and thirteen-year-old clients with this problem. In their case, a low-fat, high-carbohydrate diet will cause them to gain fat no matter what the calorie count of the diet may be. When we become insulin resistant, it's impossible to lose weight without the right combination of foods. At this point the chemistry of the diet is more important than the calories.

Metabolic Syndrome X

Insulin resistance is also known as metabolic syndrome X. This is an identifiable metabolic disorder that makes it difficult for the body to burn fat. This condition is usually due to an overexposure to highly processed types of carbohydrates. With metabolic syndrome X, the body loses its ability to regulate its blood sugar levels because the cells of the body no longer respond to insulin by taking up glucose. In other words, the body cannot get the sugar out of the bloodstream. When this occurs, the individual will begin to suffer high or low blood sugar levels, thus becoming hypo- or hyperglycemic.

Over the last couple of decades, it has become apparent that the same health problems that result in heart disease are found in those suffering syndrome X. The basic problem is the inability to remove sugar from their bloodstream, thus increasing their levels of insulin. When insulin levels are high, we are insulin resistant, and this will cause a series of complications.

Fat burning is a biological process that the body cannot accomplish when insulin levels are high. When we enter the second cycle of health as young as thirty-five years of age, our bodies become more insulin resistant, preventing our body from using fat as fuel.

Insulin versus Glucagon

There are hormones that make your body burn fat, and then there are hormones that will shut down the fat-burning process. Insulin's counterbalancing hormone is glucagon. Insulin shuts off fat burning while glucagon turns on the fat-burning response. Insulin and glucagon are two of the primary hormones involved in storage and release of energy in the body; these hormones must balance each other out for optimal energy levels and fat burning.

When we eat carbohydrates, insulin drives our metabolism to store excess food energy for later use. Glucagon drives our metabolism the other way, allowing us to burn stored fat for energy during physical activity, working, or sleeping for hours after we have eaten.

Glucagon is the hormone that releases our stored fat to be used for energy. The challenge we have is that glucagon is available to us only when insulin is not present. Insulin and glucagon cannot coexist in the body at the same time. The excess insulin produced by high-carbohydrate and low-fat diets causes insulin resistance, thus shutting down glucagon and fat burning.

In diagram 6 and 7 you can see the effects of insulin versus glucagon in the body.

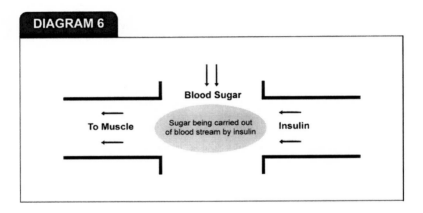

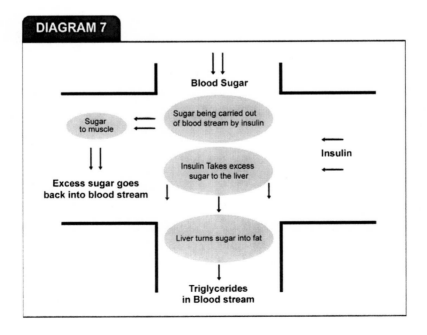

Insulin	Glucagon
1. Encourages the kidneys to retain salt and fluid.	1. Releases excess fluids.
2. Stimulates the production of cholesterol by the liver.	2. Lowers the cholesterol levels
3. Increases triglyceride production and levels.	3. Lowers triglyceride production and levels.
4. Thickens the muscular portion of the artery walls, increasing the risk of heart disease.	4. Sends signals to the artery wall to relax, thus lowering blood pressure.
5. Promotes excess body fat storage especially around the waist, hips and buttocks.	5. Burns excess body fat, reducing your waist, hips and buttocks.

Table 1

Our diet has to be balanced not only with the right foods for our particular metabolism, but the foods we consume have to be the right combinations.

2. Hormone Deficiencies

I discussed the different hormones in chapter 5, "The Cycles of Health," especially when we enter the third cycle at age forty-five. When our hormones are out of balance, it's virtually impossible to get our body to burn fat for energy. Hormones are the messengers that communicate every function that takes place in our body. Your hormones regulate your immune system, your metabolism, your energy production; hormones even regulate your moods. The balance of your hormones determines your quality of life.

Most doctors, when evaluating patients, don't put much emphasis on hormones. Rarely will a doctor check your hormone levels as part of your yearly physical exam. This is why I emphasize patient education; it's so important to get informed. I belong to different organizations where I can receive continuing education on a regular basis. I also read everything I can get my hands on, and I work with some of the best scientists and doctors in the preventative medicine field. Here are a few great books to get you started.

1. *The Schwarzbein Principle* by Dr. Diana Schwarzbein
2. *The Type 2 Diabetes Breakthrough* by Dr. Frank Shallenberger
3. *Ultra-Prevention* and *Ultra-Metabolism* by Dr. Mark Hyman
4. *Perfect Balance* by Dr. Robert Greene
5. *HRT: The Answers* by Dr. Pamela Wartian Smith

These are just a few of the countless number of books on hormones and hormone balance. I also recommend that, once you start understanding the importance of hormone balance, you find a physician that will listen to you and work with you to help you attain your particular balance. I belong to a great group that can give you a list of doctors, www.worldhealth.net or www.acam.org. These sites can get you started on your own research.

When we hear the word *hormone*, we automatically suppose that we are referring to the sex hormones. More often than not, it's not the sex hormones that are hurting our metabolism, it's usually the stress hormones, which I will discuss in detail in the next chapter. Our fat cells release several hormones that determine if we store or burn fat. Balance is determined by lifestyle and the stress-response diet will give you the blueprint to keep your lifestyle balanced with proper nutrition along with exercise and supplementation for your cycle of health.

3. Excessive Carbohydrates

The key to achieving balance is making sure we have a healthy fat-burning metabolism. Dr. Shallenberger states in his book *The Type 2 Diabetes Breakthrough*, "More than any other single factor, resting fat metabolism is suppressed by eating too much carbohydrates." I totally agree. I have been doing different tests on clients for twenty years, and I can always tell when a client is either eating too many or the wrong type of carbohydrates. After a certain age, the body just has trouble assimilating the carbohydrates in a diet. When this happens, it really doesn't matter how many calories you eat, you are not going to burn fat unless you balance out your diet. As Dr. Shallenberger puts it, "The body's fat metabolism is being hijacked by excessive dietary carbohydrates, particularly middle- and high-glycemic carbohydrates."

This brings us to the next issue. It's not always the amount of carbohydrates that sometimes affect your body, it can also be the type of carbohydrate you eat and the time of day or night at which you eat it. In part

4, "Creating your Program," I will go into detail on this issue. For now, it's essential to understand that the combinations of foods will determine if we burn fat and if we get results or not. As we age, we will develop blood sugar intolerance, which simply means our bodies change the way they processes food, and all of these changes can be detected by simple testing.

4. Insufficient Sleep

When people have difficulty with fat burning, the one common denominator that I see consistently with each individual is the lack of sleep. Most clients I see today, as they enter the middle of cycle two (around age forty), will start having more and more difficulties sleeping. This has to do with our modern stress-oriented lifestyles, where technology can have us working around the clock. This causes the stress response to become unbalanced. When we don't get enough sleep, our body will automatically go into survival mode. At this point, the body will store fat. We will then begin to get cravings for sugar, carbohydrates, and have a strong appetite in the evening, causing us to overeat. Without adequate sleep, our bodies cannot possibly keep the stress response balanced. Remember that the body burns fat when it is balanced.

At any given time, our body is going in one of two directions. We are either breaking down (catabolic) or balanced and recuperating (anabolic). The biomarkers are influenced one way or the other according to the direction our body is going. To keep our body anabolic, we must have the right mix of diet, exercise, and sleep.

During the day, when we are pushing our bodies to perform, we experience a process called catabolism. It's when your body will do what it takes for you to accomplish the feats you have set out to accomplish on that particular day. Your body will use its raw materials for you to perform. If you need more energy, your body will produce hormones that will give you a boost. This results in a breakdown of the body, putting it into a catabolic state.

At night, our body is designed to repair itself from the day's catabolic breakdown. This is called anabolism (when our body switches direction and becomes anabolic). During our sleeping hours, particularly deep sleep, we repair the damage from the day's activities. Simply put, your body recuperates and gets ready to perform again the next day. Without enough sleep, it's impossible for our body to be healthy and be able to burn fat.

Balancing our Fat-Burning Hormones

The bottom line is our bodies are made for survival. Our survival DNA is programmed from millions of years of evolution. The challenge is, and will be for as long as we live, that our body's DNA and survival instincts will remain primal no matter how much technology advances. Our body believes it lives in a cave and there is a saber-toothed tiger at the door! As I have mentioned earlier, our body reacts to whatever signal it receives. If that signal is constant stress (catabolic), it will respond accordingly. It will store fat. Fat is our emergency fuel.

During the recuperation phase of the day (anabolic), our body balances many hormones that allow us to be able to burn fat. These key hormones are cortisol, growth hormone, leptin, and grehlin. Cortisol is the body's main stress hormone and it's in action all day long. Cortisol rises in the morning to wake you up, increasing your appetite, and gives you the energy to start your day. Cortisol balances itself out at night while you sleep and it drops while growth hormone and melatonin levels rise, thus repairing the body and making it anabolic. When we suffer from sleep deprivation, we experience hormone changes that turn our body's signals upside down. When these hormones are out of balance, our bodies biology turns on its survival mode repressing our appetite in the morning, and increasing it at night. We then overeat mainly at night, usually unhealthy foods, jeopardizing any efforts to lose weight.

Two of the main fat-burning hormones are growth hormone and leptin. Growth hormone is one of the most important hormones for our health and vitality. Growth hormone has a powerful action on fat metabolism called lipolysis. Lipolysis causes the fat cells to release their fat content for energy production, thus fat burning. Leptin is a hormone that signals the body to stop eating and to burn fat. Both of these hormones are released and balanced when we get a deep sleep. End result: *no sleep, no fat burning.*

Special Note: The sleep/obesity connection is more apparent than ever as we see stress levels rise and health drop. The "win at all costs" attitude is something I deal with every day with my executive clients. It's like a badge of honor not to sleep and to work fifteen hours a day. Besides obesity, we are seeing other problems crop up as people get less sleep, such as reflux and sleep apnea. Sleep apnea, which literally means a cessation of breathing during sleep, occurs during deep-sleep levels, causing the disruption of sleep. This pause in breathing can last from seconds to a few minutes, never letting the body balance out or recuperate. If you snore loudly at night and are experiencing fatigue during the day, I highly recommend ruling out obstructive sleep apnea.

5. Carnitine Deficiency

The key factor for anti-aging, disease prevention, and a healthy metabolism is the preservation of our muscle mass or biomarker number one. As we age, our bodies have more trouble balancing stress, thus causing a catabolic breakdown state in the body. This is when our intake in protein becomes vital for our body balance. A key amino acid from protein is L-carnitine. It plays a vital role in creating a fat-burning metabolism. Without adequate amounts of L-carnitine, it is impossible to transport fat into the mitochondria to be converted to energy. Carnitine is naturally found only in meats, so cutting this food group from your diet for weight loss is not the best choice. Anthropological studies suggest that the diet of our caveman roots consisted of two to three thousand milligrams of L-carnitine. In comparison to today's average intake of five hundred to one thousand milligrams per day, there is a deficiency of this vital amino acid. I recommend at least two thousand milligrams per day.

6. CoQ_{10} Deficiency

Coenzyme $Q_{10,}$ or CoQ_{10} for short, is the cornerstone of our body's ability to create energy in what's called the Krebs cycle. A simple explanation for understanding the Krebs cycle could be that it is a series of biological reactions that occur in the matrix of the mitochondria in which electrons are transferred to coenzymes and carbon dioxide is formed. The electrons carried by the coenzymes then enter the electron transport chain, which generates a large quantity of ATP. This is also called the citric acid cycle. CoQ_{10} is part of a critical connection in the mitochondria to complete the Krebs cycle and aid the body in producing energy and boosting our metabolism.

CoQ_{10} also is a key antioxidant that protects the body from free radical damage. It actually helps to circulate the other key antioxidants such as vitamin C and vitamin E. This process prevents the breakdown of the cell from free radicals.

People who are treated for high cholesterol with the use of statin drugs run the risk of being depleted of CoQ_{10} because the same steps that produce cholesterol in the body also produces coenzyme Q_{10}. It is essential for proper fat burning and energy production that anyone taking a statin drug supplements with CoQ_{10}. I usually recommend from 50 to 300 mg a day, determined by the results of the client's cardio-metabolic stress test (bio-energy test).

7. Dietary Fat Deficiency

When I teach clients that without adequate fat in their diets, they cannot possibly burn fat, they are completely shocked. It's been embedded in our diet culture and psyche that fats are bad. This couldn't be farther from the truth. Certain fats are essential for the body to stay in balance, thus be able to burn fat. Without the essential fats in our diet, we cannot balance our hormones, prevent lifestyle-related conditions such as heart disease, diabetes, or even lose weight.

As I explained in "Biomarker Four: Body Fat," our fat cells create a communication in our body. This communication system determines whether we burn fat or not. The fat that we consume in our diets is also important for communicating to our genes. There are certain fats that are healthy and certain fats that are deadly. Whether a fat is good or bad, it has to do with the kind of information that the fat is communicating. The type of fats and the ratio of fats in your diet determine good or bad communication, and this is what controls the condition known as silent inflammation. As we discussed in "Biomarker Four," there are two types of inflammation—silent and screaming. Silent inflammation causes a cellular breakdown and disease.

When we talk about fat deficiency, we are actually referring to the balance of fats in our diet. Both omega-3 and omega-6 fats are essential to our health. The balance of these two fats will determine the overall health and function of our body. Omega-3 and omega-6 fats perform opposite functions in the body. Omega-6 fats act to increase inflammation and help our blood clot. Omega-3 fats do the opposite of the omega-6; they work like an anti-inflammatory and decrease inflammation in the body. Both these functions must be in harmony to be healthy.

The challenge that we face in our modern-day diets is that there is an overabundance of omega-6 fats and not enough omega-3 fats to create stability. The results are increased inflammation. I will go over all the different fats and the proper ratios in more detail later on in this book.

8. Trans Fatty Acids

Trans fats have been headline news recently. They are being blamed as the main culprit in the obesity crisis. I still believe that you can't just pinpoint one single reason for the rising numbers of obesity in America. The obesity epidemic is the end result of a number of variables going terribly wrong. I will say that trans fats are definitely in the top three. Trans fatty acids were created by the food manufactures to prolong the shelf lives of certain foods. For the food industry, this was a major breakthrough. The shelf life of certain foods such as crackers, chips, peanut butters, cookies, breakfast cereals, and many others were extended without any risk of spoiling.

Trans fats are truly the most damaging type of fat. Recent studies are showing that these fats interfere with the hormones that signal our body to burn fat. Several published studies have documented that these fats actually may block the ability of the mitochondria to produce energy. The challenge that we have is that these fats are found in virtually every form of processed food that we consume. You will find them in food products under the label Hydrogenated Oil or Partially Hydrogenated Oil. Trans fats will raise the bad cholesterol (LDL) and actually lower the good cholesterol (HDL). Without a doubt, these fats will prevent the body from burning fat and cause a host of bad medical conditions.

Recently, the Food and Drug Administration (FDA) has begun to require food manufacturers to state on the labels of their foods the amounts of trans fats. The problem is that *zero* doesn't actually mean *zero*. When a label says Zero Trans Fats, the FDA will allow a little and still let the label say zero. The rules state that a value that is less than 0.5 grams or half a gram per serving doesn't have to be listed on the label. Go figure. Here are a few tips to keep you on track:

1. READ the label's contents. If you see the words "hydrogenated oil" or "partially hydrogenated oil," avoid the foods and look for healthier alternatives.
2. AVOID deep-fried fast foods and takeout. Remember, they can say, "No trans fats" as long as it's below half a gram per serving. The big fraud here is not only stating zero when it's not, but also what the manufacturer considers a portion. Study the portions of breakfast cereals and be realistic at the true amount we eat. This can really add up in trans fatty acids consumed.
3. Avoid manufactured cakes, pastries, biscuits, and pies.

Trans fats should be avoided as much as possible to have a healthy fat-burning metabolism.

9. Vitamin/Mineral Deficiency

Deficiencies in certain nutrients can prevent our body from burning fat efficiently. My opinion is that if you don't use supplements after a certain age, it's virtually impossible to keep our bodies balanced. Remember, our body can only burn fat when it's balanced. Deficiencies in B vitamins, chromium, magnesium, zinc (just to mention a few) will get in the way of optimal fat burning. Omega-3 essential fatty-acid imbalance, as we mentioned earlier, can cause insulin insensitivity and compromise fat metabolism in the mitochondria. The truth is that after age thirty-five, as we enter the second cycle of health, it takes more than just exercise and diet to balance out our fast-paced/high-stressed lifestyles. It takes the right combination of supplements to keep your individual metabolism working and balancing the stress response.

Decreased fat-burning capabilities can also be linked to protein deficiencies as well. Vegetarians are more likely to suffer from protein deficiencies and especially the essential amino acid, lysine. Lysine is abundant in animal proteins, but less in grains. It converts in our bodies to L-carnitine. Carnitine, as discussed in point number 5, is essential for the fat-burning process. Carnitine appears only in animal foods, especially red meat. Many people avoid red meat for several reasons; these people need a carnitine supplement to maintain balance. It's important to understand that any deficiency will disrupt the fat-burning metabolism and your overall health. Many of my clients are truly amazed at how different they feel when they get the right vitamins and minerals to balance their body out. (See appendix C.)

10. Stress

I believe that if you manage stress properly, you will be healthy. In today's world, stress is the number 1 issue we all deal with, no matter what our age. We cannot get rid of stress, but we can manage the stress response. The stress-response diet is dedicated to creating this balance. Without this balance, it's impossible to burn fat properly.

Part Three

The Mind

Chapter Nine

It is the nature of man as he grows older to protest against change, particularly for the better.

—*John Steinbeck*

The Mind: The Key to Optimal Health

Michael was a forty-six-year-old banker who was sent to me by his cardiologist. He had been diagnosed with elevated cholesterol and borderline hypertension (elevated blood pressure). Michael's doctor wanted him to lose at least forty pounds, or he would have to start him on medication.

Michael lived a very high-stress life. On a stress scale of one to ten, he stated he was an eleven. Michael traveled at least ten days per month on business and had many late business dinners along with a very full social calendar. Michael's biggest challenge was he basically didn't have time to take care of himself. When it came to diet, he would often skip meals or grab something on the run. The last time he was on any type of exercise regimen was when he was in college, twenty-plus years ago. Like most successful professionals that I work with, Michael's focal point was career, not health.

Michael's focus changed drastically with his visit to his doctor. He was highly motivated to begin his stress-response diet; his motivation stemmed from the simple fact that he was scared. Michael's father had died at the age of fifty from a massive heart attack. Michael's elevated blood pressure and cholesterol, along with a sharp decrease in his energy levels, was a serious wake-up call. I didn't have to convince him that he needed to change his lifestyle; he was willing and ready to get started.

Michael's first thirty days in the program were amazing; he dropped twelve pounds on the scale, and actually lost fifteen pounds of fat while gaining three pounds of muscle. Michael's doctor was equally encouraged as his blood pressure dropped to an optimal range, and his cholesterol fell sixty-five points. Michael was thrilled; he loved his new lifestyle and his new look. He was wearing a size of clothing he hadn't worn in years and looked like he was ten years younger. He didn't have any problems following his program even while traveling on business.

Michael continued to make fabulous progress for the next couple of months. In as little as ten weeks, Michael dropped twenty-five pounds of fat and gained eight pounds of muscle. His waist dropped six inches; and his health, along with his energy levels, was the best it had been in twenty years. At this point, everything would begin to change. This is when Michael informed me that he was going to take a break. He said he would take a couple of weeks off, and then he would return. I tried with all my might to talk him out of this, but he was persistent.

Those two weeks turned into six months. When Michael finally did return, he had gained all the weight back and an extra ten pounds. His doctor had started him on medication to control his blood pressure and cholesterol. Michael felt embarrassed when we sat in my office to talk. He couldn't explain what had happened; he basically just fell apart and went right back to his old habits. I surprised him with my reply. I told him, "What happened to you is normal. It's not your fault!"

What happened to Michael is common of every client I work with if they let their guard down. Anytime we try to change a behavior or habit, we have to go through a certain process. This process involves what I call *testing periods*. I discovered these testing periods in the mid-1990s. As you read in the first chapter, I am very big on collecting data. When I opened my first training center, I would have the trainers keep track of each training session by having the clients sign a dated sheet that was kept in my office. These sheets were color coded so I could tell if a client canceled, didn't show up for their session, or stopped coming in altogether. I would review these sheets with each trainer on a weekly basis to find out the status of every single client at the center. What I noticed was absolutely astounding. Each client would fall off their program at a certain point of their training, without exception. During each of the testing periods, clients would cancel, get sick, or quit altogether.

What happened to Michael, basically, was that he didn't pass a testing period essential in creating a new habit or behavior. Our habits or behaviors are literally programmed in our mind. If you change that programming, you can change your life. Michael knew that in order to keep his weight off and blood pressure down, he would have to maintain a healthy lifestyle. It truly doesn't matter what we know. What matters is what's programmed in your mind; this is what results in taking daily positive action. We must literally program the habits and behaviors that we want.

Introduction to the Mind

Americans are consumed by the quest to find themselves—to find an elusive, omnipresent state of happiness. Most people I meet believe that if they can finally lose their weight, they will then find true happiness. In this desperate pursuit of happiness, they will turn to one of the many self-proclaimed self-help gurus of the day. We are all trying in a desperate way to improve the way we feel about ourselves, to be in control of our financial situation, our children's future, and so many other things. We tend to believe that if only we had a tight grip and control of everything and everyone around us, well, we probably would be happier.

As a nation, we spend millions of dollars buying "help" at bookstores and online. We attend seminars, listen to CDs, read books, and watch TV shows. All of these aids can be helpful, but they don't represent the solution we are all seeking.

In order to achieve the goals we are striving for, we have to change our habits from the core. We have to learn to create the habits we want by understanding how the programming of our mind works. We cannot learn new habits from anyone else.

The key to self-improvement is not only setting the goals you want, but also having a formula to make them real. The *Thirty Days to Change* workbook was a book I wrote over twelve years ago. I wrote this book mainly to help my corporate clients during seminars. What I found was that anyone who was seeking true change in his or her life really needed to be able to get through the first thirty days. Thousands of people have used this simple workbook to aid them in creating new healthy habits and, more importantly, change their lives forever. The power of those first thirty days cannot be emphasized enough.

Over the last twenty years, through my studies on self-improvement and human behavior and working with thousands of individuals, I have found that the most balanced and successful people share common traits and habits. From these common traits, I created the ten success principles featured in my book *The Five Links to Permanent Weight Loss*. I know that if you can get a deep understanding on how your mind works and how to create the habits that you seek, you cannot possibly fail.

Understanding the Mind

The mind is very complex and powerful, but we can learn to tap into its abundant energy. In order to be successful, we have to create a balance between a healthy body and a healthy mind. In fact, once you truly understand how your mind works, you will be able to make life's hard times easier and life's good times even greater and be able to take complete control of your body and health.

Many people don't realize the fact that our brain controls our body's reactions. We are born with a brain that is much more complex than most advanced computers. Scientists claim that people use less than 10 percent of their brain's capabilities. Can you imagine what could be possible if we doubled its output to 20 percent?

Our brain contains as many as 100 billion cells and has the ability to process up to 100 million bits of information per hour. Our brain takes care of all our bodily functions and is responsible for balancing billions of cells through the autonomic nervous system. What I find truly amazing is that every thought we have actually has an effect on how our brain functions. Dr. John Hagelin, a quantum physicist made a great statement, "Our body is really the product of our thoughts." This observation is so powerful when it comes to any type of program to change our body. The fact is our thoughts have a profound effect on the stress response.

My first experience with the power of the mind was when I found the book I mentioned in chapter 2, *The Power of Positive Thinking* by Norman Vincent Peale. It was the first time I took control of my life by controlling my thoughts. Ever since I read that book, I have dedicated a great part of my time to working and studying how the mind affects the body.

When I became aware of how the mind can work for or against you, I began developing techniques to tap its enormous power. One such technique was the power of visualization. I picked this up during my bodybuilding days from Arnold Schwarzenegger. Arnold would talk about how he would visualize exactly how he would look for each competition. I followed his advice to a tee. I would cut out pictures of the exact physique I wanted and then paste a picture of my face on to the body. I would practice thirty minutes each night, visualizing my perfect body. I might have been born with bad genetics, but I trained my mind to help me to become a champion bodybuilder. I changed my body, my metabolism, and my attitude by understanding the power of the mind. NOTE: To me, there are few better examples than Arnold Schwarzenegger (in his bodybuilding years). When it comes to harnessing the full potential of one's mind, he was a truly incredible bodybuilder.

I have studied the influence of the mind on the body through psychology courses, books, seminars, tapes, and role models. And when I learned how to take control of my mind, I never fell short of reaching my goals and never felt out of balance. When I help a client truly grasp the power that they really do possess as an individual, they never fail to reach their goals—never.

I had many destructive habits (that I thought were normal) built into my life, only to discover that I had been programmed to have them involuntarily. We all have the potential to tap into our mind's unlimited resources, but first, we must understand how the mind works.

Chapter Ten

The Components of Your Mind

Everything is based on mind, is led by mind, is fashioned by mind. If you speak and act with a polluted mind, suffering will follow you, as the wheels of the oxcart follow the footsteps of the ox. Everything is based on mind, is led by mind, is fashioned by mind. If you speak and act with a pure mind, happiness will follow you, as a shadow clings to a form.
—*Sakyamuni Buddha*

There are three components that make up the mind. They are as follows:

1. conscious mind
2. subconscious mind
3. superconscious mind

Each of these three parts of the mind has a profound effect on the actions we take and the results that we receive.

The Conscious Mind

Our conscious mind identifies incoming information. This information is received from our senses—sight, sound, smell, and touch. Our conscious mind is the analytical part of the mind. It helps us to reason. It also serves as our center of logical thinking and gives us the power of dissertation. The major functions of the conscious mind involve learning and helping us to be realistic.

It is important to understand that it is the conscious part of the mind that gives us the power to directly change our lives. Our conscious mind is capable of holding only one thought at a time. It's not the part of the mind that will cause you to take action, but it does program the action that needs to be taken. It inputs the data into our subconscious mind so we take a desired action. Our conscious mind works like a captain of a submarine. The captain sees everything that's going on through the submarine's periscope and then relays the information to the crew (subconscious mind); it's the crew that is steering the submarine, not the captain.

It's essential to be aware of the individual functions of each part of the mind. We may know what to do to improve our lives, but what we know and the actual actions that we take are two separate factors. If our conscious mind were responsible for us taking action, we would not have any bad habits; knowing and doing are two very different things. Here is an example of how the conscious mind works.

We all know that smoking is hazardous to our health and that it causes an array of illnesses, including heart disease, lung cancer, and reduced aerobic capacity (low oxygen), and many other problems. Nowadays, it is also not socially accepted, and it has become increasingly more difficult to smoke in restaurants, public places, and the workplace. With all this knowledge and information on the hazards of smoking, why would anyone continue to smoke? The answer is because the conscious mind knows the information and the facts, but that is not what makes us take action. It's the same scenario with diet and exercise. We all know that to be healthy we need to eat right and do some exercise. What we know truly doesn't matter. Whatever is programmed in the subconscious mind is what makes us take action.

To change anything in our lives, we must educate ourselves on why the particular changes are important and needed for us as an individual. True change comes not just from educating our mind, but from changing our behavior. This is done through reprogramming our habits in the subconscious mind.

The Subconscious Mind

The function of our subconscious mind is to store and retrieve information. Our subconscious mind does not think or reason; it is the part of the mind that causes us to react and take action. Our outside actions will always fit the programming and the pictures in the subconscious. Our subconscious mind responds to its input and will stay consistent with our beliefs, values, ideas, self-image, and our particular focus on life.

Our subconscious mind is like the computer's hard drive; it's the main storage of information in the computer. It stores every moment of our lives from the moment we are born. The subconscious is an unquestioning servant of our conscious mind.

Looking at our submarine, if the conscious mind is the captain of the submarine, the subconscious would be its crew. The captain (conscious mind) of the submarine peers through the periscope and relays the orders to turn right or left. The crew (subconscious mind) receives the orders and makes the turn. The crew (subconscious mind) has no idea if the turn was right or wrong. They cannot see where they are going; they just do what they are told. But it's the crew (subconscious mind) that is taking the action, not the captain (conscious mind). The subconscious mind does not think or reason; it reacts. Our subconscious reacts to whatever it is programmed for through the conscious mind. If the input is positive, then the action will be positive. If the input is negative, then the action will be negative.

Change Your Thoughts, Change Your Life

The subconscious mind is key to all your success and failure. You control your subconscious by controlling your thoughts. When we change our programming, which I will discuss later, our thoughts automatically become productive. Here are some valuable points on the subconscious mind:

1. The subconscious mind accepts whatever your conscious mind sends it; the subconscious will not argue with you.
2. If your thoughts are good, your subconscious will project good.
3. You have the power to choose your conscious thoughts. It's your choice what you feed your subconscious. Choose health and happiness, and that's what you will receive.
4. Whatever statements you choose to say are directly loaded into your subconscious. It's essential to be accountable for everything you say. I will fail, I can't lose weight, I have a slow metabolism—these are orders from the captain, you!
5. Your subconscious cannot take a joke. It believes everything you tell it. "I'm too old to get in shape." "At my age, you just start breaking down." "I look at the cake and gain ten pounds."
6. The subconscious is always about what you choose. You are the captain of your subconscious. Choose health, choose success, choose love, choose happiness!

Now that you understand how the mind works, it should be simple to make any changes we want in our lives. If you're the captain, all you have to do is give the orders to the crew—to lose weight, quit smoking, or change any bad habit you may have. We all know it's not that simple. We have to monitor our conscious thoughts, and we have to reprogram our subconscious beliefs and values to create new habits.

The New Year's Resolution

Every year, that magic date will come around on the calendar, January 1. This is the date when we all decide to finally change our lives. We promise ourselves that we will lose weight, we will find the right relationship, make more money, change jobs, write a book; and the list is endless. Unfortunately, most of us never succeed in carrying out our goals. It has nothing to do with determination, and it has everything to do with programming. In other words, we are aware that we want to change, but we just don't understand how. You will easily know if you're stuck in a subconscious programming by taking a look at your life and your goals. If on January 1 every year you have the same goals from the previous year to lose weight, stop smoking, change jobs, etc., there is a pretty good chance you are stuck. To accomplish any type of change, you have to become the programmer of your life.

All your habits, both good and bad, have been programmed in your computer (subconscious), unfortunately much of it, without your consent. Whatever is programmed determines the action you will take on a regular basis, in other words, your habits. Your subconscious has been receiving information since the day you were born; it records every single moment of your life. Our first programmers are our parents, who passed on their beliefs and values to us by raising us and instilling their personal, cultural, and other value systems. If your household was positive, proactive, and was about becoming successful, your programming would be the same. On the other hand, if your household was dysfunctional, full of drama and negativity, you will have those same traits. Most people will follow their family traits unless they understand how to change deeply embedded habits and patterns. These programmed traits have a direct effect on the stress response.

There are many other influences on our early programming besides our parents. Other programmers are our teachers, role models, coaches, the media, television, the culture where we come from, religion, and other value systems. They influence us through individual experiences and peer pressure from childhood to adulthood. Programming from television, radio, magazines, and all the advertisements tell us what to wear, what kind of car to drive, what foods give us pleasure, and even what we are supposed to look like.

When it comes to weight loss, just watch the ads that are shown. One will tell us to go to a fast-food restaurant because you deserve a break. The next ad will then tell you to buy a pill to help you finally lose the weight. When the holidays roll around, all the advertisement you see is about having these large meals with all your family gathered at the table, (no one advertises weight loss products on Thanksgiving). The ads promote overconsumption of all types of food. In America, we have been programmed to value the notion that we need more, especially when it comes to food. We spend billions every year to lose weight, but until we understand how the mind works and how to take control of it, we will ride the diet roller coaster and be setting the same goals on January 1 every year. Advertisers know that if they can get their message to your subconscious, you will take action and go buy whatever they are selling (even if it's a Pet Rock or an Ab Roller).

The Challenge of the Subconscious Mind

Our subconscious programming is where we hold our habits, beliefs, and values. If we want to change a habit, we must change the programming. *The challenge here is that the subconscious is designed never to change.* Our subconscious is what is called homeostatic. Homeostasis is defined as a condition in which the body's internal environment remains relatively constant; it's not supposed to change. Our subconscious mind controls our body mainly through the autonomic nervous system. The autonomic nervous system is responsible for all the mechanisms and systems needed to keep our bodies alive—the beating of our heart, the blinking of our eyes, the function of our organs, our body temperature, etc. This is why our subconscious mind translates its need for homeostasis to the part of the mind that creates action. Again, this is a direct link to the stress response. Here is an example to illustrate the delicate balance of the nature of the subconscious.

Our body's normal temperature stays approximately at ninety-eight degrees. There is not much difference between the number 98 and the number 102, right? Not really. When it comes to our body's temperature, this difference represents an enormous change. The body's systems go into action to get its temperature back to 98. This can involve millions of cells for all this to happen. You don't have to tell your body to get to work; it's on automatic pilot to rebalance your entire system.

This same process influences your habits, both good and bad. The subconscious mind, where you hold your habits, is also known as your *comfort zone*. What's in your comfort zone comes easy for you, automatic. Your subconscious doesn't know smoking is bad for you. You know smoking is bad, but the truth is it doesn't matter what you know; it only matters what's programmed in the subconscious. Most of us go through life and wonder why we do the things we do. We set out with good intentions to change our lives and seem to always end back where we started or even worse off than when we began.

Breaking any habit means we have to step outside of our comfort zone to create change. Wishing for these changes just isn't enough. We do not realize that our surroundings are influencing us every day of our lives. Everything we say and do is either helping us grow or keeping us stuck in a life we wish would change. We need to monitor our conscious mind and only let thoughts into our subconscious that would empower us. As you learn how to create your own lifestyle, you will understand that you can become the captain of your ship. I will show you how to program your new habits so your lifestyle becomes automatic. But first, there is one more part of the mind I would like to discuss, the superconscious mind.

The Superconscious Mind

The superconscious mind is also referred to as God, spirit, higher consciousness, the universe, or the higher self. This is our spiritual self. It is what some of us believe to be that guiding voice or influence in our life that gives us our particular direction. This is called our intuition.

The superconscious is accessed through our subconscious mind. The superconscious mind is the source of all creativity, motivation, and inspiration. It is the exciting feeling you get when you have a new idea or when you're working on a project that you love. It's when everything that you're doing seems to work effortlessly. It is the source of all pure creativity and has access to all stored information, past and present. People, information, ideas, problem solving, all comes naturally. This is when everything in your life is at a balanced pace and everything just seems to work. Examples of people who live their lives from this special place are everywhere. From Mother Theresa who just knew what she had to do with her life despite the impossibility of her dreams to Tiger Woods on a golf course, these are two examples of accessing the superconscious. When Tiger is in the so-called zone, it's literally a work of art what he does on a golf course.

The author Napoleon Hill referred to this power as infinite intelligence. In his incredible book *Think and Grow Rich*, he states that our superconscious is the universal storehouse of knowledge. He states that when you have a pressing problem, just tap into this infinite intelligence, and you will not only receive the answer, but you will always receive the correct answer. Napoleon Hill also states that all great successes enjoyed by hundreds of wealthy men and women he interviewed over the years were achieved as a direct result of this tapping into infinite intelligence or the superconscious mind.

Getting the Power

The purpose of this book is not to convert you into being a spiritual person, but to make you believe in yourself and the power of positive focus in order to change your life. It is important to understand that there are guides and forces that science cannot explain, but also cannot ignore. From everything Gandhi accomplished to what Bill Gates has created to Thomas Edison inventing the light bulb—it's a power that is very real. It's a power that will change you and your life forever.

Every day, I personally tap into this power. I feel it when I'm training and lifting weights (that are supposed to be impossible for my age). I feel it when I'm with a client. My work flows effortlessly and I instinctively know what the person needs. Whether it's a kind word or strong motivation, I allow myself to follow my gut, and it's never wrong. When I give a seminar, I never script myself; I always know from the energy of the crowd which way to focus the talk. Everything I do, when tapping in this force, seems effortless and sheer pleasure.

The main thing I believe you need to tap into this power on a regular basis is a defined purpose for your life. I defined my purpose over twenty years ago, and I base everything I do on that definition. My purpose is to motivate, educate, and inspire people to live a healthy and balanced life. How does this work in my life? Well, first, let's take the motivation part of my purpose. I'm like a coach that will always push you to live the life you deserve and the life you truly want. I will push you to make the changes that must be made for you to reach your goals. Second, I will educate you on how to do this. It's not enough to be told to change; you have to understand how. Education is the key for anyone to step outside their comfort zone and seek true transformation. Third, inspiration is about walking the talk. I know what I teach works because the bottom line is I live it every day. If I can keep over one hundred pounds off for twenty-six years, anyone can.

I go to work every single day and do exactly what I love to do. The way I accomplished this was I created my job, my business, and my career. The BioFit Centers and the stress-response diet are my work and purpose. I am here to live it each moment of each day.

Let's take these three components of the mind and learn how we can use them in our everyday life to create the changes that we seek.

Becoming a Compulsive Overeater

When I was a little boy, I wasn't considered fat; I was "husky." A well-fed child was considered healthy, and I was definitely well fed. When I was little, like most kids, I really didn't like my vegetables. My grandmother had a system to get me to eat my peas and carrots; she would offer me a dessert as a kind of reward for choking down the vegetables. I knew if I could just get those veggies down, I would get the cake. Did Grandma's vegetable-eating system work? You bet it did! I would do anything to get those delicious desserts—even eat vegetables.

This worked well until I was nine years old. That's when a diet doctor took the desserts away, even if I ate the veggies. The challenge was that Grandma's vegetable-eating system was deeply programmed into my subconscious mind. It was an urge that I can still remember today. I had to have that dessert, and it was my reward no matter what. As you can probably guess, this is when I started sneaking food to my room; it was such a powerful programming that it still is with me even today.

Another powerful programming I was exposed to in my house was the order to finish everything on my plate no matter what. Daily, I would hear about all the starving people in Africa. My grandparents survived the great depression, when food was scarce. So to my grandfather, it was a sin to leave anything on your plate. There were times I would have to sit at the table for one to two hours because I wouldn't eat, and I was not allowed to waste food.

I am part of the baby-boomer generation, and this food-and-eating-related programming is very familiar to most people from my generation. These seemingly innocent programs derail most attempts for us to lose weight. I am a compulsive overeater. Food is my crutch in this life. It doesn't matter that I have kept my weight off for over twenty-five years. I have to work on this addiction daily, or I will fall back. It's the same addiction as an alcoholic, only it's food instead of alcohol. I have to say after twenty-five years of teaching most of the overweight people that I meet are compulsive overeaters. I created the stress-response diet programs for them and for me. I recommend to my clients who have a lot of issues with food to also seek help through a therapist who specializes with eating disorders or join a group like Overeaters Anonymous (OA). I spent many years going to these meetings. They are very empowering and they will help you to take control of your life and change your patterns.

Chapter Eleven

Creating a New Lifestyle

You have learned about the mind's different components and how they cause us to act. The question people usually ask during my lectures is, "Why is it so difficult to create a healthy lifestyle of proper diet and exercise?" Believe it or not, there is an actual reason for this, and it is all linked to the programming of your subconscious mind. Our subconscious is what causes us to take action. It is what controls the body; and it is where our habits, both good and bad, are programmed. Now, consciously, we know that by changing our diet and performing proper amounts of exercise, our life would change dramatically. We would look and feel better, increase our energy levels, and we would also be able to reverse and prevent lifestyle-related diseases such as diabetes and heart disease. *As you learned, it doesn't matter what we know; what matters is what we have programmed as our habits as determined by our subconscious.*

The programming of our subconscious starts the moment we are born. Let's review my early programming. When I was a little boy, I was never called fat; I was referred to as husky. As a child, I was always told that I needed to finish everything on my plate, and then I could have dessert as a reward for eating all my food. I was then programmed to believe that I was responsible for all the starving people of the world if I didn't finish everything on my plate. Food was my reward for just about everything when I was little, from getting an A on a test or when I would fall and scrape my knee. I learned early in life that a chocolate-chip cookie could fix just about anything. At nine years of age, everything changed as my rewards for being good (food) was changed because a doctor decided I was no longer husky, but that I was now fat.

My reward system was taken away, leaving a rather large void in my life. What would I do without my friend "ice cream" when I got sad? If I choked down my food to finish everything on my plate, what was my prize? If I skinned my knee, what would I do without my treat to make me feel better? My subconscious was programmed to believe that food was my reward, my friend, my only comfort. This programming would drive me to sneak and hide food everywhere so if I needed comfort, no one would be able to stop me. As an adult, I would go off and binge by myself. If I was sad or if I was happy, food was always there for me. For me to change this and for anyone to create change, we must reprogram our subconscious mind to create the habits we want and to empower our lives.

The Comfort Zone

Many people have heard the term *comfort zone* but don't fully know what it means. The comfort zone is in your subconscious programming. The subconscious mind's programs are the actions that you are comfortable doing, right or wrong. For instance, we get up in the morning and brush our teeth. This action has been programmed in your life since you were a small child. We do not even think about it or question it; we just do it. Brushing our teeth is part of our comfort zone. If you have ever forgotten your toothbrush on a trip and couldn't brush your teeth, you know how uncomfortable that can make you feel. That's how our comfort zone works.

When it comes to diet, exercise, and health, there are many comfort-zone programming that we need to be aware of. Here are a few:

1. The less I eat, the more weight I will lose.
2. Eating carbohydrates is bad.
3. It's normal to get aches and pains as we age.
4. Exercise is about "no pain, no gain."
5. To lose weight, we have to starve.
6. Vitamins will make me fat.
7. I have to lose weight.
8. To lose weight, I have to avoid all my favorite foods.
9. I should lose the weight first, and then start exercise.
10. Cut the fat in the diet to lose weight.
11. As we age, aches and pains are inevitable.
12. I'm addicted to chocolate.
13. I love carbohydrates.

14. Training with weights will make me too big and stop my weight loss.
15. The more I sweat, the better the workout.

There are probably hundreds of different diet and exercise programs in our minds, many of them coming from the medical field or so-called experts. The challenge is this: Our comfort zone is located in the subconscious mind. It holds our habits, beliefs, and values. What's in that zone reveals the action we will take on a regular basis. Simply put, if exercise is in the comfort zone, you will love to exercise; if not, you will hate to exercise. Changing the programming in your comfort zone isn't as easy as joining a gym. Remember, your comfort zone (subconscious mind) is homeostatic; it is designed to remain the same. Whether these programs serve your life or not, it doesn't matter to the comfort zone, what matters is only what's programmed within.

Redesigning Your Comfort Zone

Let's take a look at the early programmers of our subconscious mind. In diagram 8, we see an example of an individual's comfort zone. Many of our early programmers were merely passing to us their own programs. Many of our habits are passed down from generation to generation. As you can see in the comfort zone, most of the unconscious programming we are exposed to is not necessarily geared toward helping us lose weight in a healthy manner. When we set out to create a new lifestyle or new habits, we have to be willing to step outside our comfort zone and be uncomfortable.

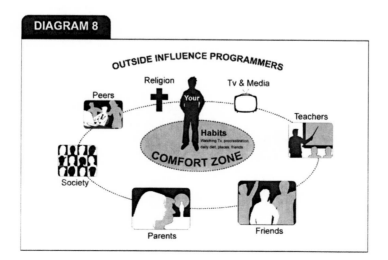

DIAGRAM 8

OUTSIDE INFLUENCE PROGRAMMERS

We have to be willing to change. This may sound a little silly, but after working with thousands of clients, you wouldn't believe what they would do to protect their comfort zones. I have seen clients who have had heart attacks and have pacemakers who would rather die than give up smoking. I have seen diabetics who refuse to manage their disease even after losing a foot. It doesn't matter how much the doctor preaches to patients to take care of themselves, they just cannot, or should I say will not, modify their lifestyle habits.

Much of this reluctance to change is related to stress. Many of our early programming was given to us during times of stress. If you hurt yourself, your mother would give you a cookie or a comfort food. If you had a bad day at school, you would probably go get ice cream. During a stressful period, we automatically turn to the programs of comfort, and our mind doesn't know if the comfort is healthy or unhealthy. In order to make real change happen, we have to get leverage on ourselves. We have to be willing to face our fears. Fear of not having dessert, of going through a holiday and not eating everything on the plate, or fear of having to exercise in front of other people or getting sore muscles—these are all fears we must face in order to grow. While you're reading this, it just may sound ridiculous, but I have to tell you, these silly fears are just a few of many that stop people from having the success, health, and the lifestyle they dream of.

The New Comfort Zone

While working in the health and wellness field over the last twenty years, I have discovered some very interesting characteristics that develop in each one of my clients as they go through their programs. Every client would have certain challenges that would come up at certain times during the first year of their program. These were very specific tests, and they were consistent in every client. The pattern was set. I discovered that over a one-year period, there would be four times in which my clients would be challenged while creating their new lifestyle. I called these times their *comfort zone testing periods*. The testing periods were times when my clients would sabotage themselves for no apparent reason, much like Michael in the story beginning this chapter. I discovered that these are the periods where the homeostatic subconscious mind wanted to return to its original programming. In other words, your habits would return to the original comfort zone. This pull is very unconscious and part of the way our mind operates; it's very powerful.

Everything in your circle is part of your comfort zone. Whatever is in this circle is familiar and comfortable in your life. Despite the substantial anxiety toward change, we have to step outside that circle in order to grow and change. Whether it is about getting healthy, losing weight, changing jobs, asking for a raise, or becoming involved in a new relationship, we have to be willing to get uncomfortable; we must take action even if we feel fear. (See diagram 9.)

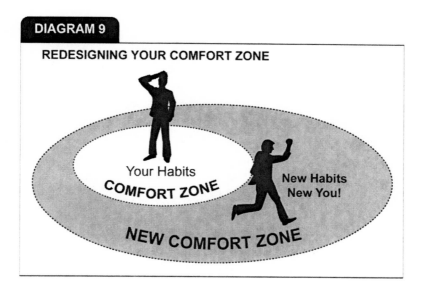

DIAGRAM 9

REDESIGNING YOUR COMFORT ZONE

Your Habits
COMFORT ZONE

New Habits
New You!

NEW COMFORT ZONE

When it comes to weight loss, many of us will stop trying as we get older for the fear of failing. If you have lost and gained weight living the yo-yo diet cycle, you may be uncomfortable with trying something new or another program. I promise you, as you will learn in the next chapter, this isn't just a program. It's a lifestyle that will give you the answers and solutions to reach all your goals, forever. Most of us are so fearful of change that we have to hit rock bottom before we stand out of our comfort zone. Confronting or challenging the limitations of our comfort zone will increase our self-esteem and confidence. I will educate you on the testing periods so you will be ready when they come. When you're prepared, you will pass these tests without any problems on your way to your new BioFit Lifestyle.

Comfort Zone Testing Periods

Your subconscious comfort zone is programmed for you to act. It does not differentiate whether the habit is good or bad. When you begin any type of self-improvement program and begin reconditioning your subconscious comfort zone, you will experience tests along the way. These tests and testing periods occur due to the homeostatic nature of the comfort zone. Just because you think or you know that change will be good for you, that doesn't mean the subconscious will consent to it.

Test One:
First Thirty Days after Starting Your Program

The first test will be obvious to you. It begins the moment you make a decision to change. Looking at diagram 9, you will see what happens the moment you take action. The comfort zone will immediately begin to kick in, attempting to pull you back to your current habits. What if I fail? What about that ice cream I have in the freezer? I'm really busy right now; maybe next week will be better. How many of us have joined health clubs and would go once and never go back? Or buy a book on change and never read it? Most of us have been through the "I'll start tomorrow" syndrome. It's absolutely normal; it's all part of the process of becoming the captain of your life.

The first thirty days present the most uncomfortable period of change. The truth is that there is only one answer that will get you through this testing period; it's *discipline*. Discipline is the answer in the first thirty days. You have to step outside your comfort zone and begin to take charge of your life. Every day, one day at a time, is the simple focus that will help you to stay on track. A great mantra to repeat over and over during these first thirty days is "discipline equals freedom!"

Test Two:
Twelve weeks from the Original Starting Date

After the first thirty days on your new BioFit Lifestyle plan, you will begin to see and feel a dramatic change in your body and health. Your life will become healthy, and your diet and exercise regimen will actually become enjoyable. In diagram 9, you see the first expansion of your comfort zone. When this expansion occurs, everything seems effortless; you follow everything without much temptation to cheat on your menu or skip your exercise.

Just when you think it's safe, you will get hit with test two, the twelve-week mark from the time you started your self-improvement journey. The challenge comes when you have just begun to make remarkable progress.

You have lost weight or quit smoking, changed your attitude, and have begun to develop a consistent routine. This is when your comfort zone homeostasis kicks in to return you to its original programming. Your subconscious wants to make sure this new lifestyle is what you really want. Remember, many of our habits have been ingrained since early childhood, and twelve weeks is not very long to reprogram an entire lifetime.

Old habits always have the ability to slip back into your life little by little. "Maybe I'm eating too much. If I cut back, I will lose more weight." (You will learn later in the book why this is totally wrong.) "I have been good, I deserve a treat." "I'm a little tired today. I will skip and start over tomorrow." All these messages are actually your comfort zone trying to return to what it believes is its proper programming.

I would like to share with you an interesting observation I have drawn over the years with this particular comfort zone test. Remember, the subconscious part of the mind controls our body. When people challenge their comfort zone, especially with diet and exercise programs, they will usually get sick around the twelve-week mark. The client will call and say they are under the weather and want to skip their appointment. Some clients actually get flulike symptoms, and immediately, they reach for their favorite comfort foods. When this happens, clients will then start making excuses to get started back on their program. From my experience, if the excuses go longer than two weeks, the client will destroy all the progress they made the previous twelve weeks by returning to their old habits.

Martha's Big Test

When I was a personal trainer, one of the things I really took pride in was my ability to keep my clients. During my training years, I had clients that worked with me for ten or more years. Martha was one of those clients I had during the 1990s when I was building the stress-response diet. When Martha started with me, I was heavy into studying the subconscious mind and the power of changing it. Martha was the first client I used the just-show-up trick on while she was going through her twelve-week testing period.

Martha was a thirty-six-year-old real estate broker that worked an average of sixty-five hours a week. Martha was around thirty pounds overweight when I met her. She confided in me that she had gained twenty pounds in the last couple of months. Before that, she thought she had found the magic diet that she could do easily without much thought. This was the great low-carbohydrate diet where she could eat all the eggs, meat, pork rinds she wanted and didn't have to worry about how much she ate, as long as she avoided carbohydrates.

When I met Martha, she was tired of yo-yo dieting and wanted to start exercising. I immediately changed her diet to balance out her body, and we started training together. Martha struggled in the beginning, missing several appointments and being late for others. After a few weeks of really pushing her to do the program, everything started to click. She was following her program to perfection, and after eleven weeks, she had dropped two full sizes and had incredible high energy levels.

When Martha hit the twelve-week test period, she started coming in late and even missed a couple of appointments. I tried to talk to her about what I was learning about the subconscious mind, but she really didn't want to hear it. Then one day, she called me to tell me she was feeling under the weather and she was going to take a break and start again next week. This is when I tried a technique to challenge her to expand her comfort zone. I simply told her no. If she decided not to come in, I would stop being her trainer. As you can imagine, she got very upset with me, yelling into the phone that she was sick. I then told her I didn't say she had to exercise. I said, "You have to show up or you lose your spot." It was no more than twenty minutes later when she stormed into the gym and confronted me with some well-thought-out words that I can't mention here. I simply told her I was so proud of her, and I would see her at our next scheduled time.

What I had learned about the subconscious was it couldn't tell the difference between dreams and reality. When Martha showed up at the gym, she was becoming the captain of her submarine (of her life). In fact, that very night she called me and apologized for her outburst, and then she thanked me. She said all her cold symptoms seemed to disappear, and she would be there for her next appointment.

"Just show up" is the best advice I can give anyone who is trying to truly create change in their life. I promise you, there will be obstacles and challenges. These are the times you truly expand your life and your comfort zone.

Test Three:
Six Months from the Original Starting Date

After six months of following the program, many clients run into a big problem—*they actually reached their goals*! For many yo-yo dieters reaching their goals is uncharted territory, and they experience complete confusion.

Can I take some time off? Can I have dessert now? Where do I go from here? This was my usual failure point during my yo-yo diet years. I would start adding in a few goodies and then a few more; before you knew, I was off and running, gaining back all my weight and a few extra pounds for good measure.

Let's focus on this issue for a moment. Once you clear the second challenge, which usually lasts from one to two weeks, you will begin to again flow at an even pace. Your subconscious believes you are truly committed to your change. What I have found with metabolic testing over the years, is that after the twelve-week test is completed, the metabolism really revs up. The clients do well until they approach the six-month mark, when again they are going to be tested. The six-month test is tricky because by this time, you have made incredible progress. You look different, feel different, act different, and everyone around you notices the new you.

Throughout all my years of working with clients, I always found this to be the hardest period in their reprogramming process. This is when you finally have made it, and all the work and sacrifice has paid off. This is when you find yourself wearing new clothes and receiving compliments from everyone. Then out of nowhere, *you begin to sabotage yourself.* A little voice tells you it is all right to miss a few exercise days or "hey, you look good and a little dessert can't hurt" or "maybe I can take an extra junk night". After all, I have been really good for six months, and I deserve a break!"

The biggest challenge many people feel during this particular testing period is that they begin to look good. People walk up to them all day long, asking, "What have you been doing? You look great!" Unless these comments are built into your comfort zone, they will make you feel uncomfortable. You are not programmed to receive so much attention. The little voice will try to convince you that you are not worthy of such praise. When someone looks at this situation from the outside, it just doesn't make sense. Here you have worked hard and accomplished your goals, you look great, yet because you're receiving attention, you feel like eating! As I'm writing this, I have to laugh because this always happened to me during my weight-loss years.

Contrary to what everyone believed about me, I was very disciplined. I would take a diet and follow it to perfection. I would lose the weight every time, then right around the six-month mark of my diet, I would hit a crazy period. I would receive so much attention that I would start to actually get angry. I would say things to myself like, "Why does everyone want to talk to me now. When I was fat no one would talk to me!" I was especially angry toward girls because when I was thin, they would pay attention to me; when

I was fat, it was as if I had the plague. I also would have anxiety about my clothes. When I would hit a certain size, I would begin to panic, and fear would set in. "What if I gain the weight back?" The results from all this pressure I was feeling were always the same. I would begin to binge because I was afraid of gaining the weight back. From the *conscious mind* point of view, this seems insane. You are afraid of regaining your weight, so you eat? This is a common theme of the six-month testing period.

This testing period is different because many of us reach our goals in this period or have made significant progress on our program. This testing period will derail every single diet out there if the diet isn't designed within a lifestyle program. If you lose weight and then go back to the same lifestyle that caused you to gain weight in the first place, you're simply going to fail! The stress-response diet is a new lifestyle, as you are progressing with your nutrition and exercise. I will give you the tools to reprogram your comfort zone. When you hear that little voice trying to convince you that you are not worthy, don't give in because you are one step away from permanent change.

Test Four:
One Year from the Original Starting Date

Test four presents itself at the one-year mark from the time you started your new lifestyle. Your subconscious programming now includes your new lifestyle habits. This is when we become the captain of our ship, and the subconscious actually works for you and not against you. This is when many people begin to refer to you as an exercise fanatic or that obnoxious ex-smoker. By this time, your exercise and nutrition routines will be part of your *new comfort zone*, and you will feel uncomfortable if you don't maintain them. At the one-year mark, your new habits are so well formed that even when you travel, you will automatically find time to exercise because if you don't do it, you just will not feel right. Now your comfort zone is your personal built-in coach, always making sure you're following your program. Now homeostasis is working for us.

I tell you, after following the stress-response diet and lifestyle program for a one-year period, very few people fall off. It becomes second nature to them; it's their lifestyle. But it is important to note that the one-year test is important to still monitor because there are circumstances that can trigger setbacks.

Betty's One-Year Test

When I share stories about my many clients, I will usually share inspirational tales of success to motivate you while you are changing your life. The truth is there are those stories of failure and heartache that also need to be told. Betty's is one such story that happened over ten years ago. She was a client that I truly loved and cared for.

Betty was a forty-two-year-old single mother of four. She was in charge of a human resource division of a large corporation with which I worked. I was creating their corporate wellness program and Betty was in charge of the wellness project I was creating for the company, so we spent a lot of time together. I had learned that Betty was recently diagnosed with diabetes, the disease that had taken her mother's life at a very young age. Betty had seen the terrible effects of the disease manifest itself through her mother, including the loss of one of her limbs, her eyesight, and finally her life. Betty was determined to take charge of her life and not let what happened to her mother happen to her.

Betty weighed close to 250 pounds when she started her stress-response diet. She had been on many diets in the past, but this time, she was extra motivated. She wanted to be the shining example of her company. During the first thirty days of her program, she was perfect. Immediately, Betty started dropping weight, and her energy and enthusiasm went through the roof. I loved watching her change and lead the entire company by example. At the six-month mark, Betty had dropped over seventy-five pounds, and her doctor had reduced her diabetes medicine by half. By the end of the year, Betty had dropped 103 pounds, and her doctor would completely take her off the diabetes medications. Betty was a true inspiration. With all her personal and professional responsibilities, she managed a perfect balance of health and corporate efficiency. But there would be an unforeseen challenge that would change everything.

Right at the one-year mark of Betty's amazing transformation, the company where she worked for over ten years was sold. This was absolutely devastating to Betty; she began to panic about her future with the new company—if there was even an opportunity for her to stay or if she was headed for the unemployment line. She was so worried she began to turn to an old friend to comfort her; that friend was food. Betty started eating totally out of control, craving foods that a week early she easily avoided. She stopped her exercise program altogether, stating she just didn't have the energy or the time to deal with it.

Betty kept telling herself she would start over next week, but unfortunately, next week never came. Her subconscious began to take her back to her old habits, to a comfort zone that had made her obese in the first place. Betty gained 125 pounds in three months. The diabetes returned, and so did all the medication. No matter how hard I tried to snap her out of this tailspin, I just couldn't.

After all, she did end up getting a position with the new company. Two years later, after many repeated attempts, she did remain obese. In fact, she was close to sixty pounds heavier than when she started the first program. Her diabetes was also out of control; her doctor finally had to start her on insulin. I haven't had contact with Betty for at least ten years, but she is a client I always wonder about. What if I had gotten her through that final test?

After a year of challenges, you will discover that you have now developed a new habit. This is when everything in your program is second nature. Your comfort zone works to help maintain your new habits. Once they reprogram their comfort zone, people who have never been athletic or who never did any type of physical activity make exercise a natural part of their life. Meeting the early challenges of the comfort zone is the key to creating any type of change that you wish.

Comfort Zone Test Summary:

- **First Thirty days**
- **Three months after starting the program**
- **Six months after starting the program**
- **One year after starting the program**

Chapter Twelve

The Comfort zone testing periods

"If you put yourself in a position where you have to stretch outside your comfort zone, then you are forced to expand your consciousness."
—*Les Brown*

Overcoming the Comfort Zone Test One
The First Thirty Days

The first step to changing your comfort zone is to understand that being uncomfortable is natural any time you pursue any type of change. Your comfort zone is somewhat like a prison that's holding you back from your dreams and goals. The comfort zone prison guards consist of can't, won't, fear, not sure, what if, and many other negative thoughts telling you not to try. For you to change your life, you have to take the first step and start. I suggest that before you start, you get prepared. Get some leverage on yourself to get you to take that first step. Here are a few suggestions:

1. Talk to your doctor about getting a wellness checkup with blood work. In appendix B, you will find the blood test that I recommend to my clients and how to read the results. These tests can reveal just how your body is working and even which phase of the program to start with. (Note: You don't need laboratory tests to get on the stress-response diet, but they can reveal a lot about how your body is currently functioning, as well as give you a comparison tool with which to measure your progress.) I also recommend that you talk to

your physician about the stress-response diet and about you following it. It would be great if you can get your doctor involved with your program.

2. Read and understand this chapter. It's the key to your long-term success. It's all right to experience anxiety when starting something new.

3. Once you are ready to begin exercising, I recommend that you find a BioFit Center facility and begin working out with BioFit-certified trainers. Most certified trainers are highly qualified but do not necessarily follow the strict exercise and nutrition guidelines the stress-response diet is based on. Remember, more is not always better, and one of the common mistakes out there is that people work out too hard. BioFit-certified trainers are taught to build personalized workouts for each individual, focusing on using exercise and resistance training to improve your health first and foremost. If there isn't a BioFit Center in your area, you can visit our Web site to download a workout you can follow in your local gym or at home.

Overcoming the Comfort Zone Test Two
Twelve Weeks after Starting the Program

The twelve-week test will usually last one to two weeks. This is the test that is essential to pass to really increase our body's metabolism. Here are a few suggestions to get through this test:

1. Be aware. Sounds silly, but the most important thing for you to do is mark this date on your calendar and get ready. Awareness is really the only thing we need. Once we know, our subconscious mind is going to act up; we will not be unconscious, and we will stay on track. It's when we get caught off guard that we sabotage our efforts.

2. If you are feeling ill during one of your scheduled exercise sessions, use the "just show up" plan. Go to your particular exercise place or check in with your trainer, and then go home. Once you get there, you may want to walk a little. Either way, you're giving the subconscious the message that you're serious about your new life.

3. Schedule an appointment with a BioFit counselor. They are trained to help you get through this test. If you don't have access to a BioFit Center, go to our Web site and click on the testing period support link.

Overcoming the Comfort Zone Test Three
Six Months after Starting the Program

The six-month test will last one to three weeks. I have found this test usually sneaks up on the individual because they become complacent. Most will have reached their goals or are well on their way. This test is really the turning point of whether you will create permanent changes or not. Here are a few suggestions to get thru this test:

1. Be prepared to hear that little voice giving you permission to cheat. Mark your calendar and remain steadfast in following your program. Honestly, most people have little trouble with this test if they are aware.
2. Do not take some time off. This is the killer with the six-month test. It's the subconscious trying to get back to its original comfort zone.
3. Schedule a follow-up appointment with your BioFit counselor, even if it's just to talk. Once you make it to six months, there isn't usually a lot of changes in your program unless you're changing cycles of health.

Overcoming the Comfort Zone Test Four
One Year after Starting the Program

The one-year test is a special one. This is when you have successfully reprogrammed your comfort zone. As you read earlier, it's still important to monitor yourself. Here are a few suggestions for this test:

1. Rejoice! Gather some family and friends and throw yourself a party or go buy yourself a gift. This is a landmark that truly should be celebrated.
2. Schedule a follow-up with the BioFit Center and do your yearly comparison. Take a look at your first tests and compare them with the new. It is truly exhilarating to see the progress.
3. Help someone else change his life. Nothing feels better than to share your success with someone who really needs your help. After one year, you will definitely know what you're talking about.

After You Change Your Comfort Zone:
How It Affects the Life around You

Accomplishing any type of goal requires you to create a new comfort zone. We all have a zone for weight, money, friends, career, etc. When we attempt to grow and we approach the edge of that zone, we will begin to feel uncomfortable. These discomfort signals can include mental tension, restlessness, or even physical discomfort. When we get these signals, we automatically begin to hold ourselves back so we can fall back into our comfort zone. When this happens, you unconsciously begin to sabotage your efforts to attain the particular goal. But what happens to your life after you have done everything right, went through the discomfort, and expanded your zone?

Sherry's New Life

Sherry was a forty-five-year-old-stay-at-home mom, who came to see me for weight loss advice. Sherry weighed 254 pounds at five foot five inches. She had been on every type of diet imaginable. Sherry had reached a point in her life where the kids were now grown, and she wanted to dedicate some time to improving herself. The first step was to get healthy again, and then she wanted to go back to school to become a teacher.

Sherry was extremely motivated; she followed every recommendation I gave her. She even did more than what I asked for, like going for walks not just once but twice a day. In a nine-month period, Sherry had dropped eighty-five pounds, and everything in her life began to change. Along with her new look came a self-confidence that no one had ever seen in her. Sherry was the type of person who would do anything for you, always putting her needs on the back burner. This was a completely different person than the woman I had met nine months earlier. She was extroverted—wearing flattering clothes, attending classes at the university, and exercising on a daily basis.

One day, she came to my office. I noticed she wasn't herself. She complained to me that she was having trouble on her diet and confessed that she had a couple of episodes of binging. Sherry also stated that she was thinking about leaving school, that she was too old. I just sat and listened, letting her just pour out whatever came up. She talked about being too busy, about how she missed the treats she used to have, how she was tired of exercising, and then finally, the truth came out. She said, "I have lost all my friends. Everyone thinks I have changed too much. They won't invite me to dinners or outings because they feel I judge them." Sherry cried, "It's not true. I never talk about my program unless someone asks."

First, I explained to Sherry this was a normal process of change. We all have to get through the comfort zone tests to accomplish a goal or make a lifestyle change, but we have to realize that there are other comfort zones we must also deal with. Every relationship we have has its unique comfort zone. At home, with our significant other, our children, our coworkers, and our friends—all have a comfort zone. When we change, we begin to affect everyone around us. At the BioFit Centers, we always see a higher success rate when couples come into the program together or when people have the support of their immediate group of loved ones and friends.

I pointed out to Sherry how lucky she was because her husband fully supported her new lifestyle and her new ventures, and that she should have a talk with her friends and ask for their support. Usually, these situations are handled by simply talking about them and by telling those close to you that what you are doing is important to you, and that you would love their support.

When we make changes in our lives, it will affect everyone around us; and sometimes, people resent this because they simply resent change. Many times, old relationships will fall by the wayside. In a way, I believe this is the universe's way to open new doors designed for your personal growth. My advice to everyone who experiences what Sherry did is to be honest with their friends, family, etc. Tell them your goals and get them involved, make them part of your plan. Many times, it may seem your spouse or best friend is trying to sabotage your efforts, and it may be true. But this is usually done unconsciously. They are literally unaware they are doing it. Communication and awareness are the simple solutions to this challenge.

It's important to recognize when these comfort zone challenges are being presented. Because they can literally drag you back to your own original zone. Remember it's OK to change and rock the boat a little in the name of personal growth.

Become the Captain of Your Ship

It is said that we change one day at a time. This may be true, but I actually believe we change a moment at a time. I believe that each moment is what actually shapes our day. If our focus is negative in the moment, the day's result will also be negative. What you think about is what you attract in life. This is how our mind is wired—the conscious relays the thoughts to your subconscious. And your subconscious causes you to act. This is called law of attraction.

The first time I learned about the law of attraction was when I read *The Power of Positive Thinking* by Norman Vincent Peale. This book really changed my life; it would be the first of hundreds of books I would study over the years while developing the stress-response diet. The other book that really set my thinking, and this program was written in the early 1960s by Dr. Joseph Murphy, was entitled *The Power of Your Subconscious Mind*. I have yet to find a better book for understanding how our mind works and how we need to work with our mind.

I would like to share with you a little of Dr. Murphy's book. From chapter 3, "The Miracle-Working Power of Your Subconscious":

> The power of your subconscious is enormous. It inspires you, it guides you, and it reveals to you names, facts, and scenes from the storehouse of memory. Your subconscious started your heartbeat, controls the circulation of your blood, and regulates your digestion, assimilation and elimination. When you eat a piece of bread, your subconscious mind transmutes it into tissue, muscle, bone, and blood. This process is beyond the ken of the wisest man who walks the earth. Your subconscious mind controls all the vital processes and functions of your body and knows the answers to all problems.

Dr. Murphy wrote this almost fifty years ago. The power of our mind is often overlooked when we talk about medicine. The law of attraction is simple when it comes to our health—what you believe, you will receive. Norman Cousins literally laughed himself back to health after being diagnosed with a terminal illness. Recently, researchers at the University of Wisconsin—La Crosse showed thirty-two runners a video about the wonders of super oxygenated water and how it could make them run faster. All the runners drank sixteen ounces of regular water, but half were told it was the super water. In a 5K time trial, the runners who thought they had taken the super water ran an average of eighty-three seconds faster than the others. By simply thinking that they had a magic drink, their exercise times improved. This is the power of the placebo effect. It's also the power of the subconscious mind.

What we focus on is what we will create. A common challenge is that our society likes to focus on the problems, and when we focus on the problem, we tend to create more problems. For example, our conventional modern medical system is geared to focus on illness; therefore, it is no surprise that we get more illness. For example, when I see a client that has been diagnosed with hypertension (high blood pressure), the focus is on the blood pressure problem and treated accordingly with medication to lower it. My focus is geared toward what has caused the client to have high blood pressure. It could be a bad diet, lack of exercise, too much stress, and a host of other things. When I get the client to think healthy thoughts, they automatically take action to create those pictures into their reality. We have a choice to focus on the illness or to focus on the cure. Whatever you choose, you will get.

I truly believe we need to really understand the power that we possess once you understand the mind and this law of attraction. I also recommend some great teachers; it's important to study daily to keep a strong conscious focus. Here is a small list of some of authors I have studied over the years and have influenced me over the years:

1. Norman Vincent Peale, *The Power of Positive Thinking*
2. Dr. Joseph Murphy, *The Power of Your Subconscious Mind*
3. Dan Millman, *Way of the Peaceful Warrior*
4. James Redfield, *The Celestine Prophecy*
5. Arnold Schwarzenegger, *The Education of a Bodybuilder*
6. Deepak Chopra, *Ageless Body, Timeless Mind*
7. Anthony Robbins, *Unlimited Power*
8. Napoleon Hill, *Think and Grow Rich*
9. Paramhansa Yogananda, *Autobiography of a Yogi*
10. Jack Canfield, *The Success Principles* and all the *Chicken Soup* books coauthored with Mark Victor Hansen

Understanding how the mind works and how to utilize the law of attraction is one of the keys to optimal health, permanent weight loss, and overall success and happiness that we can experience in our lives. Every day, I hear clients complain about how fat they are, how big their thighs are, etc. Every complaint you manifest is what you are focused on, and what you are focused on, you will receive. It's the law. You attract what you are focused on. I am getting old. I am tired. I am overweight. I am sick. I am unlucky. When you use the statement "I am," you are establishing a direct communication to the crew in the subconscious mind. Their job is to carry out the orders sent by you, the captain. I have a slow metabolism—*boom,* your metabolism slows down. I am tired—*boom*, your energy levels drop. I'm sure you get the point.

Before I close this chapter, I would like to recommend a great book on the subject of the law of attraction. *The Secret* by Rhonda Byrne. I have read literally hundreds of books on the subject. I found *The Secret* refreshing and easy to read. The part on the body really amused me because Ms. Byrne was dead-on. She talked about how we focus on weight loss. In America, we are obsessed about how much we weigh. For years, I have told clients I don't care about how much they weigh; it just doesn't matter. In *The Secret*, Ms. Byrne makes the greatest observation. If you focus on losing weight, you will attract back having to lose more weight. I recommend *The Secret* to anybody looking to make real change in their lives.

Conclusion

When people come to see me and ask me the secret of my transformation, they expect me to give them some type of dietary advice or some magic exercise combination. I tell them, "The truth is, I changed my mind." If you can grasp this simple concept of being the captain of your life, everything else falls into place. It's so easy. Manage your conscious mind by managing your thoughts, and your subconscious will figure out ways for you to succeed.

I find it empowering to know I control my health by controlling my thoughts. Your subconscious mind never grows old. Your expectations of aging as time passes causes you to feel old. You are as young as you think you are. You are as healthy as you believe you are. The mind is the key to optimal health.

Part Four

Creating your lifestyle Program

Chapter Thirteen

The basic components to create your own program

A journey of a thousand miles must begin with a single step.
—*Lao-tzu*

Introduction

Part 4, "creating your Program," is about creating your tailored stress-response diet program. You have learned in the first parts of this book how the body and mind work together to create a healthy metabolic balance. In "Creating your Lifestyle Program" we will take a closer look at the five bio-links and how to incorporate them into your lifestyle. Let's take a quick review of the five bio-links.

Bio-Link One: Meals. This is the meals bio-link of the program. Here you will learn how to create a fat-burning menu. This link is based on the understanding of our body's survival needs and the development of a proper combination of foods to create a healthy fat-burning metabolism. In this link, we will discuss the fat set point and how, by controlling it, it's possible to achieve permanent weight loss. In this link, we will focus quickly on the latest research on fat-burning hormones and the keys to keeping them balanced. "Meals" will provide you with an understanding of the three phases of menus used in the stress-response diet and a full explanation of the different foods and their proper combinations for you.

Bio-Link Two: Hydration. We have all been told the importance of drinking enough water. In my opinion, as I related in the earlier chapter on stress, without hydration, we cannot have balance. This link will educate you on the physiological importance of keeping the body hydrated to rid itself of excess fat and toxins. Hydration is also a key to increasing our metabolism. When researchers measured people's metabolic rate before and after drinking about sixteen ounces of water, they found a rise in calorie-burning capability. The water had a lasting effect as well. Even after thirty minutes, drinkers were using 30 percent more calories than those who stayed dry.

Bio-Link Three: Circulation. As I travel throughout the world teaching the BioFit program, I have found that even though people are very confused about dieting, when it comes to exercise, they are really confused. We have all been taught that losing weight is mainly about burning calories. The harder we exercise, the more calories we will burn; therefore, the better the results. You will learn that this simple equation isn't so simple or all that true. In link three, I will teach you how to take the guesswork out of your exercise routine. In this link, you will learn the importance of monitoring your heart rate in order to guarantee you fat-burning results. Improper exercise or exercising too intensely can actually slow down your metabolism and accelerate your biological aging process. Link three will give you the proper guidelines to create a fat-burning machine without the "no pain, no gain" philosophy.

Bio-Link Four: Lean Body Mass. Link four may be the magic link for turning any health problem around. In "The Body," we learned that the key biomarker to be healthy is muscle. Your muscle will determine how healthy your biomarkers are and what your biological age is. Muscle mass will also determine if you have a strong or weak metabolism. As I mentioned in the biomarkers, it's the muscle-to-fat ratio that dictates the overall health of our body. With all that said, resistance training and weight-bearing exercises are crucial for keeping and increasing muscle. I said this earlier in the book, "After more than two decades of helping people to get healthy and lose weight, without this link, its impossible to maintain any type of weight loss and overall well being." I will teach you how easy it is to fit these simple exercises into your lifestyle program, no matter what your current age and condition may be.

Bio-Link Five: Junk Night. In this link, I will be educating you on several hormones that are responsible for whether you lose weight and keep it off or lose weight and gain it back or whether you just don't lose weight at all. Basically, link five is an important key to maintaining any type of permanent lifestyle program. It's all about following your stress-response diet for six days on, and then taking a day off so we can actually reward ourselves every week with our favorite foods. Junk night works both psychologically and physiologically, which I will explain in its entirety later in the book.

Bio-Link One: Understanding "Meals"

A Quick Note on "Bio-Link One: Meals"

There is much confusion on what is the best diet or even how a diet should actually work. I have found that the clients I see are much more successful when they are educated. This is why I have divided the meals bio-link into three parts. The first one will educate you on the stress-response diet theories. The second part will break down the components of the stress-response diet and the third part will give you what you need to construct your stress-response diet menu.

Diets Alone Don't Work

Everyone I meet always asks the same question, "How does your diet work?" I give the same answer each time, "No, actually I believe diets alone don't work." It always brings a look of surprise to their faces. The bottom line is that generic diets alone do not work in succeeding at improving a person's level of health or at helping a person stay thin. Your diet has to be part of a lifestyle program that is right for your body and your particular cycle of health. If my hormone balancing diet works for me, that doesn't mean it's the right combination of foods for you too. I will give you the tools for you to create your tailored menu to help you control the stress response.

I spent almost half my life obese, trying anything and everything to lose weight. Would you agree that when it comes to choosing a diet or weight-loss program, it becomes extremely confusing? On one end of the spectrum, you have the experts telling you "don't eat fat, keep your diet high in carbohydrates, and you will lose weight." On the other end, you have a different group of experts telling you "stay away from carbohydrates, and you will lose weight." Then you have programs that tell you "buy our packaged food, and you will lose weight." Others tell you to count calories, count points, drink our shakes, or just take a magic pill. What is the truth?

Let's take a look at the facts. The diet industry started more or less in the seventies, but hit full force in the nineties. According to the Centers for Disease Control and Prevention, the percentage of the U.S. population considered obese has doubled since 1990. This is in spite of the fact that we Americans spend billions of dollars each year on weight loss. Last year alone, it is estimated that Americans spent over $35 billion on different programs. Now let me ask you, if those programs worked and the $35 billion actually bought answers and results, what would the weight loss industry sales projection be for the next year? Well, you would naturally think that it would be less, but no, the projections for next year are higher. In fact, if we don't make some kind of change, obesity may overtake smoking as the number 1 preventable disease in the United States.

We are learning more every day on just how complicated it actually is to lose weight and keep it off. There are dozens of hormones that must be balanced to burn fat efficiently. Most of us have been taught that to lose weight, we have to burn more calories than we consume. It's just not that simple. Here are the five keys to unlock your fat-burning metabolism.

Five Keys to Burning Fat and Creating Permanent Weight Loss

1. Stop trying to lose weight. I tell every client I see: "your goal and focus should not just be to lose weight, but to lose excess fat in a way that will allow you to keep it off." Sounds like common sense, right? No, how does the diet industry measure your progress? By how many pounds you've lost. How does the doctor measure your health? By how much you weigh. These are both wrong as we discussed in part 2, the biomarkers are the key to how strong your metabolism will be. The key biomarker is muscle. So if I drop twenty pounds off you on the scale and those twenty pounds happen to be muscle, what have I done to you? Yes, you are twenty pounds lighter; but I have just accelerated your biological aging process and destroyed your metabolism. You must focus on losing inches. Focus on losing sizes in your clothing, and you must focus on feeling great. You will know when you're on the right menu and that your body is burning fat because you will have great energy, no cravings, and you will never be starving.

2. Eating the proper combinations of foods at the right time of the day. If you want to see a perfect metabolism in action, just take a look at a baby. They wake up screaming for food, and they repeat

the act every three to four hours. The timing of your meals become just as essential as the food you eat. It's all about the signals we are giving our body. I will give you the proper combinations of food you need to promote fat burning and a balanced metabolism.

3. Supplement what your body needs to create balance. The key to longevity, disease prevention, wellbeing, and permanent weight loss is the body's ability to use fat for energy. The challenge here is that the body cannot burn fat if it's out of balance. This is where supplementation can make all the difference. When we take supplements, we need to take what our body needs to balance itself out. In my case, I have trouble processing sugars, so I need to use chromium to aid my body's metabolic process. Along with the stress-response diet, supplementation can increase effectiveness. It's important to understand what you personally need. I will discuss this issue later in the book.

4. Understand your body's need to survive. I talked earlier on this issue of the body's survival mechanism when it came to stress. It's essential to remember that our bodies are not designed to exist in today's hyper-speed, multimedia, and omnipresent-technology environment, so our natural cycles are being thrown off. Our bodies are programmed for survival and will react to whatever signal it receives. I will discuss this in further detail later in this chapter. Understanding our survival instincts as humans is key to controlling our health and weight.

5. You must manage stress and the stress response. As I discussed earlier, I believe that stress is the number one cause of obesity today. Corticosteroids, such as cortisol, are stress hormones that are part of the body's fight-or-flight system of survival. High blood levels of corticosteroids trigger storage of abdominal fat. Fat is stored to help the body deal with physical dangers such as fighting predators or other humans. Cortisol breaks down the body's biomarkers and throws the cell's energy balance off, causing us to crave sweets and calorie-rich foods so the body can store more fat. Cortisol influences food intake and metabolism through its effect on several other hormones such as insulin, leptin, and neuropeptide Y (NPY). When these hormones are out of balance, this will cause binge eating especially at night. It's just your body's way of storing more energy to survive. The stress-response diet is all about managing these hormones. The bottom line is, if we don't manage the stress

hormones, our body's cells cannot burn fat for energy and that breaks down the biomarkers and destroys our metabolism. This management is incorporating all five bio-links in the stress-response diet. If one link is missing, you break the chain of health.

The Body's Will to Survive and the Fat Set Point

One of the very first things I learned about dieting is that it's impossible to diet, lose weight, and keep it off. I learned early in my career that my diet failures had nothing to do with me, but had everything to do with the diet itself. Long before the fat-burning hormones were discovered, I learned about the *fat set point*. This was a huge discovery for me because I stopped blaming myself for my many weight-loss failures. Today I know much more about losing weight and keeping it off, but the one key in those early days was understanding the *fat set point theory*, and I want to share it with you as it really helped me understand why diets really could never work. In my first book, *The Five Links to Permanent Weight Loss*, this was the foundation of my early programs.

You have to realize that your body is an amazing self-adjusting machine designed for survival under the most extreme conditions. Your fat set point is one of your body's survival mechanisms. It is a gauge your body uses to adjust its metabolism and body weight according to the signals that it receives.

You must accept that the amount of fat that you have on your body is what it believes it needs, according to the signals that your body gets on a regular basis. Fat is not some evil curse that is put on our bodies so we have something to complain about. Fat is simply stored energy that our body believes it needs for our survival and our fat set point regulates it.

We all have a fat set point gauge in our autonomic nervous system. This is the system that keeps our hearts beating, lungs breathing, cells working, and everything that takes place in our bodies without us consciously doing it. Our fat set point is embedded in our survival DNA. Our early ancestors experienced *times of feast* in which they had plenty of food and *times of famine* when they had very little food to go by. The body had to learn to adapt to these conditions in order to survive.

Today, we live in a supersize culture where the amount of food we waste could probably feed many other countries. There is no need for this feast/famine survival mechanism; the chances of starvation setting in are remote at best unless, of course, we go on a diet. This is where our lesson begins.

As we learned in part 3 "The Mind" there are two parts of the mind that play a key role in our metabolism, the *conscious mind* that knows and is aware of reality and the *subconscious mind* that is mainly programmed by our daily habits. The subconscious cannot tell the difference between dreams and reality. Our subconscious programming is what causes us to take action, and our subconscious is what controls our body. Our fat set point is located in our subconscious mind; this means that consciously, we may know that we are overweight, but our body believes that our current weight is correct because of the past signals the body has received.

The Fat Set Point In Action

Isabel's Story

Isabel was a thirty-two-year-old bank executive and single mother when I first met her. She was a master at juggling her career and being a proactive mother for her daughter. Needless to say, Isabel's stress levels were quite high. And with her busy lifestyle, her health began to decline. She had gained more than forty pounds of weight in the five years since the birth of her daughter. Isabel had done all kinds of different diets over the years; she would lose ten or so pounds very quickly and then become so overwhelmed with cravings and anxiety she would binge and gain back all the weight plus a few extra pounds. Obviously, by the time I met Isabel, she was completely frustrated with the whole diet thing and was ready for a change.

I explained to Isabel, as I have to thousands over the years, that her diet failures were not her fault. It's impossible to diet, lose the weight, and keep it off. It has to do with our built-in survival mechanisms over millions of years of evolution. We cannot force our bodies to change by not feeding them and beating them through intense exercise. I tested Isabel and formatted a program of nutrition and exercise that could fit into her busy lifestyle. In a matter of five months, she had lost thirty-five pounds of fat and gained five pounds of muscle, and she was actually wearing a size smaller than before she had gotten pregnant. She accomplished all this without anxiety, cravings, and hunger.

Let's take a look at how our body reacts to a regimen of forced weight loss. Let us say you are fifty pounds overweight with a weight of two hundred pounds. You have maintained this weight for a while neither going too much up or down. This would establish that two hundred pounds would be where the gauge is set. This would be your fat set point.

You decide it's time to get back in shape and lose the weight. You have made up your mind that this time you will make it work and stick to the program no matter what. At first, the diet is hard, but then it becomes relatively easy. You lose the first twenty pounds quickly, and you're thinking, *This time, I will succeed.* Then it happens, seemingly in a moment, everything starts to change. *For anyone who has ever dieted, think back to your last diet program when this happened.*

1. You start getting fatigued. Your energy levels drop, and you become listless and less motivated in your daily activities.
2. You start having uncontrollable cravings for sweets and fats. It gets to the point where the only thing on your mind is food, usually junk food.
3. Your moods begin to change. You get irritable, impatient, and even the smallest thing will set you off.
4. Your weight loss stops. You're struggling and fighting to stay on your diet, but the scale doesn't move at all. You get stricter with the diet, cut back further on your food intake, and the scale doesn't budge. In the diet world, this is called a plateau. In the real world, this is usually the beginning of the end.

These are the *four signals of famine.* This simply means that the body thinks it is in a state of starvation. During my diet years, every time I lost weight, I would hit a point where no matter what, I couldn't take the diet anymore. When this point would hit, I would start craving foods that I normally wouldn't crave if I weren't on a diet. I would always crave cheeseburgers—not just any cheeseburger, it was always McDonald's cheeseburgers. I swore when I hit the famine point, I could spot those golden arches from miles away. Here's the kicker: I don't even really like McDonald's cheeseburgers, and the only time I wanted them was when I was on a diet.

What happens when the body hits that plateau and gets into a state of famine? When you lost the first twenty pounds, you were on top of the world celebrating your new body, feeling like a million bucks, right? Wrong! The scenario usually plays out something like this. We have a bad day at work, and our stress levels are high. We leave work and get stuck in traffic for an hour or more. All this time, the stress is increasing along with your cravings for a chocolate-chip cookie. By the time you get home, you're completely exhausted, and the only thing on your mind is that cookie.

You get into the house and you begin a round of negotiations with yourself. "I have lost twenty pounds, I deserve at least one cookie." After you finish the entire bag of cookies, you call Domino's for a pizza and then you have a dessert and so on—all the time telling yourself, "I will start my diet again tomorrow." Anyone who has ever been on a weight-loss diet knows that once this starts, *tomorrow never comes*. It's the beginning of the end of another diet program. Let's take a closer look at what actually happened.

1. We start a diet and the fat set point in our example was two hundred pounds. This means that the body believes it has to weigh two hundred pounds in order to survive, even though in the example this person is fifty pounds overweight. Remember, your body never knows that it is overweight.

2. The body weight drops down from 200 to 180 pounds. The signal the body receives is famine. The body now believes it's starving to death. We know consciously that we are not starving to death; in fact, in our example, this person still has thirty pounds to lose. Remember that our bodies are controlled by the subconscious mind and the signals it receives. In other words, it doesn't matter what you know, what matters are only the signals the body gets—and the signal is there isn't enough food (famine).

3. The body's job is to survive, in other words, its job is to get the body weight back up. So the body begins to sabotage our willpower to force us to hunt for food by kicking in the famine signals. Famine signals: fatigue, cravings, mood swings, decreased metabolism.

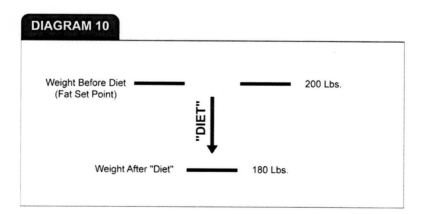

DIAGRAM 10

Weight Before Diet   ━━━━   ━━━━ 200 Lbs.
(Fat Set Point)

"DIET" ↓

Weight After "Diet"   ━━━━   180 Lbs.

5. The body's signals finally overwhelm us, and we break down and start eating uncontrollably. This is called a binge. A binge can last a day to weeks, and no matter how much we want to stop eating, we just cannot. Basically, this is the homeostasis response of the body returning to a state of balance.

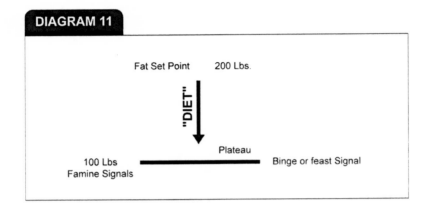

6. After a prolonged eating spree (binging), the body will begin to balance things out. Your hunger signals will return to normal and you will stop eating, but you will have regained all the weight that you had lost. The problem here is that since the body received the starvation signal (famine), the body will react by adjusting its fat set point. The bottom line is, after each diet, you gain the weight back plus an extra five pounds. With the fat set point now higher, it becomes more and more difficult to get to a normal healthy weight.

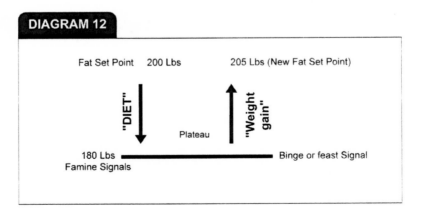

Our bodies are programmed to survive, and every signal the body receives has a cause and effect. Most people believe that the less they eat, the more weight they will lose. This theory of consuming less food causes many people to skip meals, reasoning that they will lose more fat over time. French researchers found that this isn't true. They recruited twenty-four subjects—twelve who were used to eating three meals per day, and twelve who ate four meals per day. They changed each group's meal frequency to that of the other group. The experiment lasted one month, and the biggest changes happened to the group that decreased their number of meals from four to three. People in the decreased meal group gained body fat and increased blood leptin levels (a crucial weight-controlling hormone). The other group showed very little change. This was a small experiment, but it stays true to the results I have seen over the last twenty-five years of testing my clients. If we try to force our bodies to change through severe calorie restriction or bad eating patterns, our survival instincts will kick in. The fat set point is built in us to keep our weight at the level that our body believes it needs to be for survival.

Diets and accelerated aging

Your body is an amazing self-adjusting machine designed for our survival under the most extreme conditions. When it comes to weight loss, our machine (body) always perceives this as a dangerous sign that we are in trouble. Automatically, our body will adjust to the lower calories by adjusting its metabolism. When this survival mechanism kicks in, we will decrease our health and increase the aging process of the body by breaking down the biomarkers. This is the reason that it becomes harder to lose weight as we age. When we are young, dropping five to ten pounds was as easy as starving ourselves for a few days. As we get older, weight loss becomes even more frustrating especially after years of yo-yo dieting. The years of dieting will increase our biological age because of the loss of muscle mass. When you diet, you lose three things:

1. Water. The first thing to go on a diet is our water. So when the scale begins to drop quickly, it's not fat loss that is causing it; it is loss of water.
2. Muscle. Muscle is the second thing we burn on a calorie-restricted regimen. This happens when the signal of famine or starvation

triggers the body to go into survival mode by shutting down its metabolism.
3. Mind. The final thing you lose is your mind. This is when the signal of famine will drive you to overeat (binge).

You see that the one thing we don't lose on a diet is FAT. Our body, as you learned in part 2, "The Body," only burns fat when it is healthy and balanced. When the body gets out of balance, the body's job is to store as much survival fuel as possible. You guessed it—FAT.

Lowering the Fat Set Point

Our early ancestors' main problem was keeping the body fed. There would be times of feast when there was plenty of food, and then there would be times of famine when there was little or no food available. The body would adapt to the conditions in order to survive. Today, most of our survival DNA is no longer needed. With all the modern luxuries, we have plenty of everything (especially stress). But the challenge is that our bodies have no idea that we are living in the year 2009 or 2010. Our body still thinks that there is a tiger outside the door, and it reacts accordingly to whatever signal it may receive. Stress signals the body to fight or flight, and dieting signals the body to go into "famine," causing a metabolic slowdown and increase storage of fat.

It can be tricky to lower our fat set point; it's the reason why so many diets fail. The stress-response diet is designed to give our bodies the proper signals to burn fat. When you lower your fat set point, wonderful things begin to happen to your body. Inches will disappear off your middle and anywhere you have excess fat, and you will have higher energy levels. To lower your fat set point, you must give the body the signal that it doesn't need its current amount of stored energy (fat). This is accomplished by giving the body the signal that it has plenty of live energy (food), creating the signal of feast.

The signal of feast is accomplished by eating at regular intervals throughout the day. *When the body is in feast mode, the signals it receives are that there is plenty of live energy (food) and there is no need to store energy (fat).* When your body continually receives the signal that there is plenty of live energy (food), then it will not have a need to store extra energy (fat), thus lowering your fat thermostat (fat set point). This is what allows you to achieve permanent fat loss without any of the famine signals that we discussed earlier.

Creating Your Metabolic Furnace

When feasting (eating on schedule), you are creating a *metabolic fire* that burns fat and gives you an abundance of energy. Digestion is one of the body's most effective calorie-burning activities. More than exercise, digestion causes the body to increase its metabolism in order to process foods we have consumed. When creating your metabolic fire (fat-burning metabolism), you will need to create a consistent signal of feast. In other words, for you to build a strong fire (metabolism), you have to keep fueling it. *This metabolic fire starts with breakfast.* Breakfast is defined in the dictionary as a meal eaten in the morning. A closer examination of the word is "to *break* the *fast,*" meaning breaking the night's fast with a meal, this is essential. Our bodies are designed to rest and rejuvenate every night; this is accomplished through a period of fasting while we sleep. Upon awakening each morning, we must give the body a signal of feast—that there is plenty of live energy by eating (breakfast). The fact remains that without breakfast, it is impossible to balance the stress response.

Most clients, when they first come to see me, are not hungry in the morning, so they skip breakfast or eat too little to establish a strong metabolic reaction. I have found that there are two reasons for not being hungry in the morning.

1. The stress hormones and the stress response are out of balance. When we have unmanaged stress, we usually have an excess of adrenaline. Adrenaline is the hormone that gives us energy to fight or flight. When the body is in this state, it's on a survival schedule. So stopping to eat is not high on the body's priority list. This is how diet pills work. They increase adrenaline in the body; this causes your heart to race and shuts down the hunger response. *Note: When you take these pills, it throws the body more out of balance, causing loss of muscle mass. These pills speed your heart rate and can destroy a healthy metabolism, and in some cases, can be fatal.*

2. The body's signals are in famine; it simply doesn't believe there is enough live energy, so it shuts down the hunger mechanism and slows the metabolism. The cycle of famine throughout the day throws

the body upside down. So now you're starving at night, and this is when you will eat with a vengeance.

When your body is healthy and the stress response is balanced, you will awaken in the morning wanting a good breakfast, and you will find at night, you're not very hungry. These are the signals of a balanced metabolism:

- Hungry in the morning
- Less hunger at night
- High energy levels throughout the day
- No cravings for sweets

How Often Should You Eat?

After consuming breakfast and kick-starting your metabolism, the fire has started. The trick after this is to give the body a consistent signal that there is plenty of food available (feast). By fueling the body at regular intervals, you build the fire of your metabolism ever higher. We need to eat every three to four hours to keep the body healthy and balanced, especially if you have high stress levels. In "Bio-Link One: Meals," you will learn the phases of the menu and the exchange lists. But the truth is you can actually eat a perfect combination of foods, and if you don't eat on a proper schedule, you will not be able to burn fat or balance the stress response. This is especially true as we enter the second cycle of health and beyond.

In part 3 of this link, you will learn how to set your schedule and the tricks you need to know when you have to travel or are in meetings. Consistency is the key to a healthy lifestyle and strong metabolism. Our bodies are run by our subconscious mind and the signals it receives. Lowering your fat set point is all about sending the right signals. Here are the points to lower your fat set point:

1. Always start your day with a balanced breakfast.
2. Do not miss your meals or snacks; you must maintain a proper schedule. You actually have to eat to lose.
3. Remember your body is run by the subconscious mind, and it reacts to your signals. You may consciously know that when you skip breakfast, you are going to eat lunch; but your body doesn't know that, and it will automatically slow down.

Chapter Fourteen

Hormones and Weight Loss

When health is absent, wisdom cannot reveal itself, art cannot manifest, strength cannot fight, wealth becomes useless, and intelligence cannot be applied.

—*Herophilus*

Contrary to popular diet beliefs that claim that in order to lose weight, you must simply eat less and exercise more, I am here to tell you that it just isn't that easy. The focus has to be about *burning fat* over just losing weight. To burn fat, our body has to be in a state of homeostasis (balance), and there are some key hormones that go along with the stress response which are involved in this process. Our body's ability to store excess energy for the future was critical for our survival when food supplies were scarce. Now that we live in a world of abundance, our body's signals have gone a bit haywire. Let's take a look at some of the key players in this process.

The Leptin Hormone

In 1994, scientists discovered what they called the leptin hormone. scientists were studying the ob/ob mouse. This particular mouse is three times bigger than the average mouse. Scientists found that this mouse was larger because it was missing the hormone leptin.

Leptin is responsible for sending a signal to the hypothalamus (in the brain) to cue the fat cell to release fat to be used as fuel. Leptin also acts like a signal that regulates hypothalamic neuropeptides, which in turn exert control over appetite and energy balance. Basically, leptin is responsible for shutting down the hunger signal in the brain.

When scientists administered the leptin hormone to the overweight mice, they immediately began to lose weight. Scientists thought, "Oh, my God! We discovered the cure to obesity." Well, it turned out they were right, and they were wrong. When these same scientists began to administer the leptin hormone to overweight humans, they did not react in the same manner as the mice. The administration of leptin in humans did not result in weight loss.

The reason for this is that humans, unlike the ob/ob mice, have the hormone leptin in their system. The management of stress and the person's lifestyle, including proper nutrition and exercise, directly defines the leptin levels and leptin's ability to accomplish its purpose.

Despite the disappointment that artificially administered leptin did not result in fast fat loss, scientists realized the crucial role leptin plays in promoting fat loss and how to create the right conditions for leptin to function, thus resulting in true weight loss.

The stress-response diet is designed with its five bio-links to create proper signals to balance your natural leptin levels in order to allow your body to metabolize fat as a source of fuel.

How Leptin Works

Leptin is a hormone secreted by fat cells contained in white adipose tissue, the undesirable fat that accumulates around the abdomen, buttocks, and thighs. The leptin hormone experiments demonstrated for the first time a physiological system whereby fat cells produce a *hormonal signal* that directly came from the fat cell itself. The more triglyceride a fat cell contains, the more leptin it generates. The brain responds directly to this signal by altering appetite and energy expenditure. This discovery of leptin gave us a completely different view of our fat cells. We now know that our fat cells send messages that directly control our body fat metabolism.

Leptin is one of our body's survival hormones. This hormone directly supports the fat set point theory. This theory, as we discussed earlier, is a gauge that controls and monitors our weight and the amount of fat we have. When the body perceives a calorie deficit (fewer calories) whether through diet or exercise, leptin levels will drop. Within two to three weeks of steady low levels of leptin, a signal is sent to the hypothalamus in the brain. The brain believes that the body is starving and behaves accordingly by promoting hunger and energy conservation. These, once again, will kick the body into survival mode, causing the four signals of famine to appear. These signals are also representative of an imbalanced stress response.

1. Increased Cravings
2. Mood Changes
3. Decreased Energy
4. Decrease in Basal Metabolic Rate (Slower metabolism)

When all these factors take place, the body will simply go into hibernation and become catabolic, burning lean body mass and storing fat. Other hormones as well, especially stress hormones, affect leptin. I will discuss this later.

Maintaining Leptin Balance

In order to maintain a healthy leptin balance, we must have a balanced lifestyle program. The stress-response diet provides you the tools to create and maintain a healthy lifestyle that will keep your body balanced. What we learned in part 2, "The Body", is that before we can create health, we have to balance the body's hormones, and leptin may be one of the most important to balance.

It is said that leptin is responsible for the balance and regulation of many other hormones in the body, such as the thyroid, adrenal, pancreatic, stress, and sex hormones. When leptin is out of balance, it causes obesity, immune deficiencies, bone loss, gastrointestinal problems, liver problems, cognitive problems, heart disease, and even cancer. Leptin is also responsible for carrying the messages from the hypothalamus to the fat cells to inform them that it is OK to release its fat storage to be used as fuel.

When we gain weight, the fat cells release more leptin, which is designed to make you eat less and help you burn more calories to regulate your fat set point (normal weight). This process also works in reverse. When you lose weight (body weight drops below the fat set point), the cells will release less leptin to signal you to eat more to balance out the body's reserves for energy. The challenge begins when the communication between the leptin hormone and the brain fails.

If this communication is cut due to an excess intake of fats and processed carbohydrates or too much body fat (obesity), the body becomes confused. The body is producing an abundance of leptin, but the connection is lost; and the brain stops sending the signal to use fat as fuel, and instead, continues to promote fat storage. In other words, you can weigh nine hundred pounds, and it doesn't matter what diet you are on; if leptin communication is disrupted, fat loss cannot occur. I know this from firsthand experience.

When I was obese, I really didn't eat that much. I find the same to be true with some obese people I have worked with at the centers. I am shocked at how little some of them actually eat. Most times, medical professionals think these patients are not telling the truth. I can tell you it is true that many obese people actually eat way below their metabolic rates. Leptin resistance sends a consistent signal to the brain that there is too little leptin, and the brain sends the signal of famine, starvation, and promotes more fat storage; this creates the cycle of obesity. Even if the individual is obese, the body believes it is starving. Is it any wonder why diets don't work?

The Hormone Connection

What I have found over the years is that when any hormone is unbalanced, the body will not burn fat properly. Leptin is the only fat-derived hormone with a definitive action shown to participate directly in regulation of fat stores. But there are many other groups that have an effect on fat burning.

Adiponectin

Adiponectin is a molecule produced and secreted exclusively by fat cells that normally circulate in the bloodstream. In obese individuals, it has been shown that adiponectin levels are lower. Adiponectin has been shown to help insulin pull sugar from the bloodstream into the cells where it can be converted into fuel or stored as glycogen. The fatter you are, especially fat accumulated around the middle, the less adiponectin your body will secrete. This will cause the body to have more trouble processing carbohydrates, causing insulin resistance. The main issue that prevents fat burning is insulin resistance. It seems adiponectin may play a critical role in this process.

Gut Hormones

Appetite reflects a very complex system that has been created by our bodies to help us deal with the cycles of feast and famine. Our body is built with the tendency to store fat for survival. Scientists are currently discovering a growing list of gut-derived hormones that are responsible to give signals to the brain when there has been enough food.

Three of these gut hormones are *cholecystokinin (CCK), peptide YY$_{3-36}$ (PYY)*, and *ghrelin*. *CCK* is released in the upper gut in response to breakdown of products of digestion. It is important to relax and chew our foods well to help get the signal of satiety to the brain so *CCK* can decrease the appetite. *PYY* suppresses the desire for food intake for extended periods of time. *PYY* is an excellent candidate for a future weight-loss drug. In 2005, the New England Journal of Medicine reported that PYY reduced appetite in both obese and normal-weight people. The subjects consumed 30 percent less food at an all-you-can-eat buffet after receiving the hormone compared to those who just received saline. *Ghrelin* is a hormone that stimulates appetite, and levels are particularly high immediately before a meal. This is the opposite response that you get from PYY. Obese individuals tend to have elevated ghrelin levels when they try to lose weight. When people go on a calorie-restricted diet, ghrelin levels will rise even higher.

Most weight-loss drugs in development are aiming to control these hormones. Gastric bypass surgeries aim at, not only limiting the volume of food a person consumes, but also to alter the gut hormones that cause appetite and satiety. I have worked with hundreds of patients that have had this procedure, and my main challenge is that they don't eat. They literally have zero appetite, so I have to put them on a strict schedule to prevent malnutrition.

Stress Hormones

We have already gone over the stress hormones and their role in fat metabolism. As I stated before, I believe that unmanaged stress response is the main cause of obesity and most health problems. Manage the stress hormones; manage the metabolism. The way I see it, it's rather a simple explanation. Fat is our survival fuel when we have unmanaged stress, the body will increase fat storage for its own survival. In other words, when we are stressed out, for instance, standing in line at the bank, the body cannot tell the difference between that stress or something really life threatening, it just reacts. Thus, we store more fat.

Insulin and Glucagon

I discussed these two hormones in detail in chapter 9, "What Prevents Fat Burning?" These hormones work in conjunction with each other. They must be balanced in order to properly burn fat. Insulin is the power hormone of the two, and insulin determines the balance of fat burning. Managing insulin levels is essential to overall health. Insulin is one of the most anabolic hormones in the body, and it's one of the keys to maintain our muscle (biomarker one). But excess insulin can promote cancer cell growth as well. The obesity epidemic is linked closely to insulin resistance, which increases blood sugar and insulin levels. Many researchers believe that the increased incidence of insulin resistance and diabetes will trigger more cases of cancer in the future. Type 2 diabetics have an increased risk of cancers of the colon, breast, liver, and pancreas. A seventeen-year study of twenty-nine thousand male smokers in Finland showed that men with the highest insulin levels were twice as likely to develop pancreatic cancer as men with lowest levels (JAMA, 294:2872-2878, 2005)**2. This long, extensive study shows a direct link between lifestyle and degenerative diseases such as cancer, heart disease, and stroke. The stress-response diet and lifestyle program is the best way to prevent insulin resistance and its repercussions.

The Bottom Line on Hormones and Losing Weight

When our hormones are out of balance, we will not burn fat efficiently. I have discussed many of these hormones throughout the book. Here is a quick list of others, and I am sure these are just the tip of the iceberg:

1. Estrogen/Progesterone. It is estimated that estrogen has four hundred crucial functions in a woman's body. These include increasing metabolic rate, improving insulin sensitivity, maintaining muscle (key Biomarker), improving one's mood, etc. Most women experience weight gain after entering menopause.
2. Testosterone. Males experience hormone changes and weight gains the same as women. Testosterone is an important hormone for males and females. Testosterone increases and maintains muscle mass (biomarker one), decreases excess body fat, and gives a person a sense of well-being.
3. DHEA (dehydroepiandrosterone). This has been called the mother of all hormones. DHEA is released from our adrenal glands. It converts

---

**2 *JAMA, 294:2872-2878, 2005. Finland, JAMA. Insulin, glucose, insuline resistance. Pancreatic Cancer in male smokers.*

to other hormones such as testosterone, estrogen, and progesterone. The main function of DHEA is to help the body deal with stress. DHEA production starts to drop in our late twenties, and I believe it's what causes many of the changes that we experience when we enter the second cycle of health at age thirty-five. In this cycle, the body doesn't react to stress the same way and starts to break down. By age seventy, we only produce one-fourth of the amount we made in our twenties. I have tested individuals in their early thirties showing extreme low levels of DHEA. These individuals were always under extreme stress. Most of the clients I work with that have been diagnosed with fibromyalgia, a disease tied to stress, had low levels of DHEA. DHEA has been shown to decrease triglycerides, stop the damaging effects of stress, improve sleep patterns, and increase sensitivity to insulin, plus increase muscle and strength. *A word of caution*, even though DHEA is an over-the-counter supplement sold in every supplement and drug store, you should never take it without having your blood levels checked. When DHEA levels are too high, it can also throw all the other hormones out of balance, and high levels have been linked to potential cancer cell production.

4. Thyroid Hormone. An imbalance of your thyroid hormone can affect every metabolic function in your body. Your thyroid acts like your body's thermostat. The thyroid modulates everything from fat metabolism, digestion, vitamin uses, and even our moods. These are just a few of the functions of our thyroid. Our thyroid function starts in the brain where thyroid-stimulating hormone (TSH) is made in our pituitary gland. This hormone is sent to our thyroid gland to make T_4 or thyroxine. T_4 is converted to T_3 in the liver or kidneys and is called triiodothyronine. The key for a healthy thyroid function is this conversion to T_3. T_3 is five times more active than T_4 and is a key for a healthy metabolism.

5. Melatonin. Melatonin is a very important hormone when it comes to burning fat because it sets your twenty-four-hour cycle. Melatonin is the key hormone for sleep and to balance out serotonin, a hormone connected to good mood. When melatonin rises, serotonin will fall, allowing your body to get proper sleep and recuperate. When this hormone is out of balance, you will suffer from sleep deprivation. When your body cannot process carbohydrates properly, you will make less melatonin because carbohydrates shift your amino-acid balance to make serotonin. Melatonin is a key hormone for sleep,

immune function, and stress balance and stimulates the natural production of growth hormone.

In conclusion, achieving permanent weight loss can seem almost impossible. Actually, it's quite easy once you get the body balanced. My entire career has been spent working with many doctors to help my clients achieve balance. It's important after age thirty-five to get the right testing to see what's right for you. The stress-response diet is geared to help you create a balance with your survival mechanisms, such as your fat set point, and a balance with your hormones. The main hormones that we must keep balanced to burn fat and lose weight are the stress hormones. The good news is that these hormones usually can be balanced through a proper lifestyle of diet, exercise, and supplementation. The stress-response diet will give you the blueprint to succeed.

Chapter Fifteen

Bio-Link One: "Meals": Understanding the components of your Stress Response Diet

"To eat is a necessity, but to eat intelligently is an art."
—*La Rochefoucauld*

Our diet is key to what we look like, how our clothing fits and the key to our quality of life and our longevity. While Americans' life expectancy has increased more than seven years for men and more than six years for women from 1960 to 2000, a 2008 study from Harvard Initiative for Global Health, for the first time, showed a drop in certain areas of the country. In some areas, particularly parts of the South and Appalachia showed a decrease in life expectancy of four percent in men, and one in five women. This is despite the advances in medicine and the medical field.

These recent findings can be directly connected to the so-called American lifestyle. Since the late 1970s, the number of overweight children has grown from 5 percent to 13.9 percent for ages two to five. It has gone from 6.5 percent to 18.8 percent for six- to eleven-year-olds, and from 5 percent to 17.4 percent for twelve to nineteen-year-olds. According to an article from the Harvard Medical School in 2003, adult obesity has climbed to 31 percent (59 million people), meaning they are thirty or more pounds over their healthy weight, and 65 percent are either obese or overweight or ten to twenty pounds over their healthy weight. Obesity is linked to numerous diseases from heart disease, diabetes, to different types of cancer. With these statistics, the future for America's health-care system is greatly at risk.

Everyone is given the same simple solution to fix the obesity problem, eat less, and exercise more. After twenty-five years of working in this field, I will tell you it's not that simple, but it is actually easy if done right. My conclusion after working with thousands of clients from around the world is that if we manage stress, we will lose weight. Stress is an area that isn't given a lot of consideration when it comes to obesity and disease. I have found that if I can manage the stress hormones, the body will respond with a stronger immune system, more energy and weight (fat) loss.

Every client I see tells me that stress is one of his or her major concerns. I recently did a seminar for a group of students ages ranging from twelve to fifteen years of age. When I asked them how many were under a lot of stress, 90 percent of the class responded yes. We cannot change the fast-paced world we have now created and the stress that comes with this pace, but we can manage it through our lifestyle. Through the proper menu that allows the body to balance the stress response, proper exercise that keeps our biomarkers healthy, and learning to monitor our thoughts and understanding how our mind works, we can easily get into shape and live longer.

Stress and My First Bodybuilding Contest

In 1984, I competed in my first bodybuilding competition, Mr. Central Wisconsin. There were two different competitions—one was the novice contest for beginners, competing in their first competition, and the open competition for those who had competed before. I had decided to enter both competitions that day, not really expecting a whole lot of success in the open show, but I wanted the experience.

I was in great shape for the show, having followed a regimen created by my coach that involved twelve weeks of rigid dieting with hours of cardio and posing practice. I was training three to four hours a day. The person who coached me was an ex-champion himself and was very honest with me about having expectations. He made it clear that because I didn't use any steroids, I could have a chance in the novice competition, but no way could I win the open.

The day of the competition, I was so nervous that I was physically sick. The novices were up first, followed by teenagers, women, couples, and then the open men's class. I prepared backstage, pumping lightweights and doing isometric exercises; but my physique was looking much different than the day before. The day before the competition, I was vascular (veins were showing) and very cut (the muscles were showing). No matter what I did, I couldn't get that look back. I went on to take fourth place. Onstage, I was so nervous that I was visibly shaking as I posed. I was very disappointed with the results because I knew I was better than fourth place.

After the novice competition, I had a good two to three hours before the open competition would start. I went back to my hotel and fell into a deep sleep. After I awoke, I felt refreshed and very calm. I didn't have any expectations of winning the show; I was just going to do my best. I went through the same ritual backstage, pumping up and getting ready. I didn't pay too much attention to my physique because I really didn't believe I had a chance to win.

When I stepped onstage, my coach almost fell over. I looked better than I had the day before. I was cut, vascular, and most importantly, relaxed. Between rounds, my coach came to me and told me he couldn't believe how my body had changed, and that I could actually win the competition. In the end, when the winners were announced, I had won the open class. The difference from the novice to the open was that I simply relaxed, and my body responded. This was when I really started focusing on the stress response and the body. That was twenty-four years ago, and I have never forgotten the role stress played in that competition.

The Chemistry of a Diet

One of the keys to creating health, managing the stress response, and losing weight is the daily diet we consume. Most nutritionists and weight-loss experts are consumed with the amount of calories a diet has. My experience is that the chemistry of a diet is more important than the amount of calories. When we eat the proper combinations of food for our individual metabolism, and we eat at the proper times for our lifestyle, we will create balance in our body. The main balance, as I have said throughout the book, is the balance of the stress response; and giving the body what it needs to recuperate, manage the stress response, and stay anabolic. When we have this balance, the body easily uses fat for its energy needs. When this fat burning occurs, the following happens:

1. You will have very sustained energy levels throughout the day. When we are imbalanced, we have energy levels that go up and down.
2. You will sleep more soundly. You will not have to force the body to sleep; it will naturally wind down at the end of the day to sleep and recuperate for the next day.

3. You will be able to concentrate better and think more clearly.
4. You will not crave sweets or carbohydrates. You will also find that you have a limited hunger at night. Simply put, you will not get home at night starving and craving.

When all these factors are in play, you simply don't have to worry about calories, you will not have the urge to overeat. It's when we don't properly manage our stress that we get cravings, overeat, and easily store more and more fat for survival.

Quick Reminder

Before we get into the menu construction and the foods, I want to take a moment for a quick Reminder from the section "The Mind." Science has proven that the mind plays an important role in the chemical operation of compounding and transforming food into required substances to build and keep the body in repair. When you experience worry, excitement, or fear, this will interfere with the digestive process. When you have these negative feelings and thoughts, you cannot create a harmony of digestion, thus not managing the body's stress response.

It becomes obvious that if we eat with our mind occupied with problems, our digestive process is interfered with. In this state of anxiety, we will tend to eat quickly, causing us to overeat because the brain cannot receive the signal "that's enough food!" When digestion is interfered with, the body cannot get and process the nutrients it needs to maintain balance and health. This process will cause many diseases to manifest themselves.

We talked in "The Mind" that our thoughts have a direct response on how our body functions for better or worse. The stress-response menu will give the proper combinations of foods to create harmony in the body, but an even more important key to health is the harmony of our thoughts and mind. I will give you quick eating tips to accomplish this when we construct your menu.

The Components of the Diet

There is much confusion on which food groups are healthy and which food groups you should avoid. The truth is everyone's diet has to be tailored toward his individual physiology and his particular lifestyle. Also, as we change through each cycle of health, the way our body processes foods will also change. For you, as an individual reading this and doing this program, your success will be determined much by your understanding of what and why each food group is essential to the balance of your diet. This education allows you to understand why certain combinations and choices need to be made to create a perfect menu for you.

Protein

The Key to a Healthy Biological Age and Managing the Stress Response

Protein is essential for the body to maintain its muscle mass. Muscle is the key to having healthy biomarkers. Without adequate amounts of protein in your diet, you cannot keep the correct body composition in order for the body to be anabolic. When it comes to managing the stress response, protein is key to whether or not you will keep your body balanced. Protein is not only essential for the muscle, but also it is essential to maintain your brain, bones, and vital organs. Protein is also the key to maintaining a strong metabolism and weight management.

Protein and carbohydrates have a very similar calorie count, but a very different effect on the body and its metabolism. The type of food we eat, whether it is protein, carbohydrates or fats, has different reactions and effects on the liver where it is processed. What truly affects our bodies is not the calories of foods we eat but the way they impact our bodies and our metabolisms in the process of digestion, and what effect they have in our overall chemistry. When we have balanced chemistry, we will not be hungry and will not have cravings, and thus we will not overeat.

The liver is the metabolic factory of the whole body. It's the most important organ because it regulates the use of calories for energy. When carbohydrates or fats are ingested, the liver doesn't need to change these substances very much before they can be used in the body. Carbohydrates and fats increase the liver's metabolic rate by only 4 percent. On the other hand, protein is a very complex calorie. Proteins form the backbone of the genetic signaling system. Everything in the body is made up of protein. The liver must take proteins from food and assemble them into various needs for the body. Without adequate protein, the metabolism sits still.

Believe it or not, I find most of my clients after age forty are not usually close to eating the amount of protein they need in order to be balanced. Without the right amounts, types and timing of protein in the diet, especially after the second cycle of health (thirty-five to forty-five years of age), the body cannot recuperate from the breakdown caused by *stress* and is unable to maintain the body's muscle mass, thus deteriorating the biological age and the health of the body.

Most of my clients after age forty try to become a little more health conscious. This is usually the first time they will actually go and get their first complete physical evaluation. Their doctors will usually tell them that they have to cut fat from their diets and start exercising to prevent heart disease and diabetes. The dietary changes they make when they try to cut fats out results in cutting their protein intake dramatically. They cut out eggs from their diet, and they begin to eat what they call heart smart cereal and juice for breakfast, salads for lunch, and finally, at dinner, they get their first serving of protein. There is no way in today's fast-paced world that the body can create balance on a diet without adequate protein. Remember earlier, we discussed the number one factor that increases the breakdown of the biomarkers (muscle) is stress. It's this simple, stress breaks down the body. What repairs the body? Protein!

When an athlete is training hard for an athletic event; as the intensity of the training increases, so will their protein intake so they can recuperate. The business executive over age forty-five who is working twelve-hour days with numerous deadlines is no different from an athlete. They both need to recuperate from high levels of stress. Protein is one of the keys for stress management and balancing the stress response.

Protein Misunderstood

Many people, especially medical professionals, have the impression that a diet high in protein is bad for you. Kidney damage, liver damage, heart disease, osteoporosis, and others have all been blamed to some degree on high protein intakes. In 2001, the American Heart Association (AHA) and their nutrition committee made this statement, "Individuals who follow high protein diets are at risk for . . . potential cardiac, renal, bone and liver abnormalities." From personal experience and much testing of thousands of clients, I have not seen this evidence of health problems when we increase our protein in our diet. Actually, most scientific data is now saying the opposite—that increased protein is actually healthy for the body. Protein forms the structural material for most of your body. It is essential that your cells get enough protein, especially animal protein, to make muscle tissue and repair damaged organs. Proteins are the building blocks of brain neurotransmitters. They also produce enzymes, hormones, and are practically involved in all aspects of the body.

Kidneys

The kidneys are involved in nitrogen excretion, and thus, it's been theorized that a high nitrogen intake (protein) may cause stress to the kidneys. When patients suffer from renal disorders, the standard recommendation is a low-protein diet to protect the kidneys. To conclude that a high-protein intake damages the kidneys can be very questionable. A study examining bodybuilders with protein intakes of 2.8 grams per kilogram (a kilogram equals 2.2 pounds) versus well-trained athletes with moderate protein intakes revealed no significant differences in kidney function between the groups.

Additionally, a review of the scientific literature on protein intake and renal function stated, "There is no reason to restrict protein in healthy individuals." Furthermore, the review concluded that not only does a low-protein intake not prevent the decline in renal function with age, it may actually be the major cause of the decline. This would be caused by the breakdown of muscle and the biomarkers. One of my clients who suffered from renal cancer was following traditional treatments and dietary recommendations (low protein) and his body began to deteriorate very quickly. After going to an alternative nutritionist, who immediately increased his protein intake to five times a day using supplements between meals, he started to regain strength. While he started getting stronger by increasing his protein intake, his laboratory tests showed no problems with his kidney function.

Heart Disease and Diabetes

One key to prevent heart disease is to get the lipid panel (cholesterol) under control. Traditionally, it has been about lowering the intakes of fats and cholesterol in the diet. My experience after reviewing thousands of lab results is that a diet low in fat and cholesterol rarely makes a difference in the levels of blood serum cholesterol.

It's mainly when I increase the protein in the person's diet, add more healthy fats, and lower the carbohydrates that I see the results change. When I put our clients on the BioFit phase two menu—40 percent carbohydrates, 30 percent protein, 30 percent fat—we see fast changes. I have personally seen cholesterol drop fifty to sixty points in one month. The reason is that this combination of foods will drop the triglycerides down and help raise the HDL good cholesterol and lower the VLDL, thus lowering the bad cholesterol (LDL) and improving your health and risk factors.

This diet ratio of foods is great to control, and in many cases, it reverses the effects of diabetes. The latest research indicates a 40-30-30 menu was superior to the traditional diet of 55-15-30 (carbohydrates, protein, fats) in maintaining glucose homeostasis, increasing insulin sensitivity and improving glucose control in normal people and those suffering from type 2 diabetes.

Weight Loss

When it comes to weight loss, diets higher in protein have consistently shown better results than those with higher carbohydrates. When our diet lacks in protein, we will begin to crave sweets and more carbohydrates in general. Without adequate protein, our bodies cannot repair themselves, throwing the stress hormones out of balance and causing the body to store fat.

Almost everyone knows that to lose weight, your energy intake must be less than your energy expenditure. Most nutritionist have been taught that calories determine weight loss and not necessarily the type of calories you consume. Several well-controlled studies have shown that in diets that are high in protein and lower in carbohydrates, the participants lose more weight than the standard higher-carbohydrate menu. The researchers speculated that high-protein meals suppress appetite better than high-carbohydrate diets, causing people to eat less. From my personal research, the reason why these diets work is because they help the body to maintain healthy sugar levels, and they manage the stress hormones so the body doesn't become catabolic. The key is to get the right combinations of food at the right times of the day.

Participants in a study published in the American Journal of Clinical Nutrition reported greater satisfaction, less hunger, and weight loss when their protein intake was increased to 30 percent of the calories consumed. The participants in this study ate some 441 fewer calories a day when they followed the higher protein regimen. Another study reported in the Journal of Nutrition showed that a high protein diet combined with exercise enhanced weight and fat loss and improved cholesterol levels.

"Our research suggests that higher protein diets help people better control their appetites and calorie intake," says researcher Donald Layman, PhD, a professor at the University of Illinois. "Diets higher in protein and moderate in carbohydrates, along with a lifestyle of regular exercise have an excellent potential to reduce blood lipids and maintain lean tissue while burning fat for fuel without dieters being sidetracked with constant hunger."

It's a fact that when a person increases their protein intake, they will lose fat and be less hungry. The reason for this is because they give their body what it needs to balance the stress response. When I have clients over the age of thirty-five years, who don't take protein snacks between lunch and dinner (around 3:00-4:00 p.m.), they always lose muscle when we test their body composition on their follow up appointment. When they miss their snack, they will also complain of cravings for sweets and find themselves very hungry at night. This is due to the imbalance in their stress response.

How Much Protein Do We Need?

The recommended dietary allowance (RDA) for protein is fifty-six grams a day for men and forty-six grams a day for women. I can tell you for a fact that these recommendations are not even close to what a busy executive or housewife with kids needs to balance the stress response. Dr. Layman's research recommends 120 grams of protein per day to get the potential weight-loss benefits. Layman states, "There are no dangers associated with higher intakes of protein unless you have kidney disease."

I agree with Dr. Layman. I know that to lose weight, we have to have adequate protein intakes. The reason is because to lose weight, we have to control the stress response, and without protein, the body cannot recuperate. Stress is stress; it doesn't matter if it's due to sports or a board meeting, the body still breaks down and needs to be repaired.

In the stress-response diet, I recommend 100 grams of protein split in five meals throughout the day for a woman and 125 grams in five meals for men. It's important to take in adequate amounts of protein throughout the day. Protein recommendations change with different lifestyles. For example, if you exercise often and with increased intensity, I usually recommend one gram of protein per pound of body weight. For some athletes, I recommend even more protein; it depends on the individual and the amount of stress they have in their life.

Fats

One of the most widely misunderstood food groups over the last fifty years has to be fats. We have been bombarded by the notion that if we want to be healthy and lose weight, we must cut out the fat in our diet. When we eat low-fat foods, we can actually create fatty-acid deficiencies. We have all heard how saturated fats cause heart disease and increased cholesterol levels. The truth is we actually need saturated fats and cholesterol to maintain healthy tissues, cell membranes, and hormonal balance. Cholesterol and saturated fats from such forbidden foods as eggs, coconut oil, and lean meats are actually an essential part of a well-balanced diet.

We have been taught in the last thirty years to replace saturated fats with healthier omega-6 polyunsaturated fats. Reducing the diet of saturated fats and increasing polyunsaturated fats such as corn oil, canola oil, safflower oil, and other vegetable oils actually can create an imbalance of the body, and many of the diseases that we see today. We get plenty of omega-6 essential fatty acids in our diets from milk, grains, seeds, vegetables, and most packaged foods we consume. A diet high in polyunsaturated fats can actually promote heart disease, cancer, decreased brain function, and immune system dysfunction. The reason for this is *increased inflammation*.

Inflammation

Silent inflammation is caused by an imbalance between omega-6 polyunsaturated fats and omega-3 polyunsaturated fats. According to Dr. Barry Sears, author of *The Anti-Inflammation Zone*, there are two types of inflammation. One is screaming inflammation when we injure ourselves. Here, there is visible swelling and redness and pain. It hurts. The inflammation we are addressing here is called silent inflammation. This inflammation is what destroys the cells in our body. Research indicates that the effects of silent inflammation are the basis of aging and age-related diseases such as diabetes, cardiovascular disease, some forms of cancer, Alzheimer's disease, autoimmune diseases, and obesity.

When we have silent inflammation, our cells cannot function properly or produce energy from fat. This leads to the breakdown of the biomarkers, and the body can no longer react to the stress response properly.

Inflammation and Fat Hormones

We discussed in "Meals" the fat hormones. Scientists are realizing that excess body fat doesn't happen just from overeating. They have realized that the fat cell communicates and is actually an active endocrine organ. Fat produces hormones, as do our pancreas, thyroid, parathyroid, adrenals, pineal, pituitary, testes, ovaries, and the organs that comprise the endocrine system. When we have silent inflammation, the fat cell that communicates and determines how much fat you store gets thrown off.

With elevated inflammation, our fat cells lose their ability to communicate with the body. This communication is what affects our appetite, our energy expenditure, and our immune system and how our body handles the stress response.

Controlling Inflammation:
Managing Fat Ratios and Insulin

To control silent inflammation, you must follow the proper lifestyle. There is no magic pill, and it comes down to proper menu and combinations of food. It's about monitored exercise, it's about supplementation, and it's about preventing inflammation by controlling the stress response. One of the first lines of defense is the ratio of our essential fatty acids.

Omega-6 and Omega-3 Ratios

Omega-6 and omega-3 are essential fatty acids that need to be consumed in our diet or supplementation because our body cannot produce them. The relationship between these two omegas is critical because they self-check each other in a delicate balance to regulate thousands of metabolic functions through prostaglandin pathways. Nearly every biological function is somehow interconnected with the balance between omega-6 and omega-3. Omega-3s are closely involved in the control of inflammation. The balance between these omegas is what determines the balance of the body's inflammation process.

The relationship between the omega-3, eicosapentaenoic acid (EPA), and omega-6, arachidonic acid (AA), is particularly important as the ratio of these two fatty acids is what will determine if you are experiencing silent inflammation. EPA is involved in the anti-inflammatory process in the body while AA is involved in the proinflammatory process. Adequate levels of omega-3 fatty acids, docosahexgenoic acid (DHA) and EPA in particular, have proven effective against age-related diseases such as heart disease. In addition, when you have a healthy ratio of AA to EPA, it has been shown to improve conditions such as fibromyalgia, rheumatoid arthritis, asthma, and diabetes. I have also found that when I balance a client's fat ratios that they will lose weight easily without hunger.

EPA represents omega-3 status and is involved in the anti-inflammatory process. AA represents omega-6 status and is involved in the pro-inflammatory process. The balance of these processes is what determines our long-term health. Inadequate omega-3 intake coupled with excessive dietary intake of omega-6 fatty acids can result in elevated AA to EPA ratios and silent inflammation.

During prehistoric times, humans evolved on a diet of approximately 1:1, AA (omega-6) to EPA (omega-3) ratio. The average American diet ratio is said to be anywhere from 10:1 to 50:1 ratio of AA (omega-6) to EPA (omega-3). In other words, in the best case scenario, most people consume more than ten times more inflammatory omega-6 fatty acids than required. This is one of the major causes for the obesity and health problems that we are facing today.

The Ratios and the Impact on Our Health

Heart Disease. According to the 1994 Lyon Diet Heart Study, a Mediterranean diet, which had a 4:1 ratio of omega-6 to omega-3, was associated with a 70 percent decrease to cardiovascular mortality compared to the American Heart Association diet, which has a 14:1 ratio.

Diabetes. A diet with a 20:1 ratio of omega-6 to omega-3 is associated with increased incidence of diabetes. Where as a 6:1 ratio is associated with decreased incidence of diabetes.

Rheumatoid Arthritis. A 2:1 or 3:1 ratio of omega-6 to omega-3 is associated with a reduction in arthritis symptoms. I have personally witnessed these same types of results in my clients with fibromyalgia.

Obesity. We understand that obesity causes inflammation; fat cells produce cytokines that produce inflammation. This is a lot like the chicken-and-egg theory, which comes first, the inflammation or obesity? The solution is a diet that will allow the body to burn fat. Reducing fat reduces inflammation, and that increases every aspect of your health.

Insulin's Role in Inflammation

Insulin is responsible for regulating the amount of sugar in our bloodstream. This is because insulin plays a distinct role in inflammation.

High blood sugar causes glycation and will cause a spike in insulin that increases the pro-inflammatory eicosanoids, which inflame the body and create silent inflammation. As we discussed earlier, managing the stress response is about managing three hormones cortisol, adrenaline, and insulin.

Because fats are higher in calories, most experts have been recommending low-fat diets for the most part of the last few decades. The idea has been that the lower the fat, the better the weight loss. This philosophy leads to a proliferation of low-fat food products in the market place. These foods were low in fat, but heavy in carbohydrates and sugar. Their high sugar content would cause a quick rise in insulin; and then a large drop, leaving the consumer with low insulin and severe cravings for more sugar. This rising and dropping of insulin causes inflammation and fat to increase seemingly overnight.

Most overweight people I see have elevated insulin levels and elevated inflammation. We know that to get them healthy, we need to lower their insulin levels so they can lose fat and lower inflammation. So you would think the solution is to cut out the carbohydrates, right? Wrong! As overweight people start to cut out their carbohydrate intake, their insulin levels will begin to drop.

When this happens, there is a catch-22; as insulin levels decrease so does inflammation, which allows the body to utilize fat for energy. This all seems to be right. However, as we discussed earlier, insulin is a hormone required to bring protein into the cells to maintain muscle mass (biomarker one). The overweight person has cells that are insensitive to insulin (insulin resistant) due to its chronic high levels. The body cannot recognize the new lower levels of insulin, thus it's unable to trigger the amino-acid uptake needed to maintain muscle mass and the ten biomarkers (this is why low-carbohydrate diets don't work in the long run). The breakdown of the biomarkers causes a domino effect that increases biological age and decreases our overall health.

The stress-response diet program is designed to prevent and reduce silent inflammation. The stress-response diet menu is designed to give you the right combinations of food at the right time to keep the body balanced. The stress-response diet program also gives you the other vital key to reverse and prevent chronic inflammation, and that is proper exercise. Over exercising can put you into a catabolic state and increase inflammation. The right exercise, though, can help your cells to start functioning properly, thus reducing inflammation. More on this later.

Measuring Inflammation

Many scientists and doctors are now acknowledging the role of inflammation and disease. Many physicians are now measuring C-reactive protein (standard test at the BioFit Centers), a marker of inflammation to identify patients at risk for heart disease. This test is as important as cholesterol and is actually proving to be a better indicator of potential cardiovascular disease. In fact, many cardiologists now report that elevated C-reactive protein is four times more accurate in predicting heart disease than elevated cholesterol.

C-reactive protein is a special type of protein produced in high amounts by the liver during episodes of acute inflammation. High circulating levels of C-reactive protein also indicate stomach inflammation. Researchers at UC Davis found that endothelial cells (the delicate lining of the circulatory system) also produce C-reactive protein, a key finding that helps explain how plaque formation is initiated. Researchers also found that elevated levels of C-reactive protein can cause these endothelial cells in our arteries to produce a substance called plasminogen activator inhibitor, which can lead to blood-clot formation and the potential for sudden emergencies such a stroke or aneurism. C-reactive protein can also lead to activation of white blood cells in the lining of the arteries to promote plaque formations creating blockages. This is why excess body fat causes increased risk of cardiovascular disease.

Scientists have discovered that excess weight leads to low-grade chronic inflammation and an elevated C-reactive protein. British researchers in a ten-year study showed a direct relationship between increases in body weight over time and increases in C-reactive protein levels. They measured C-reactive protein and body weight in 1,031 adults in 1990 and 2000. The average person gained nearly 6.5 pounds and C-reactive protein increased by 30 percent. C-reactive protein sensitive test is a test I recommend to all my clients yearly. It's an important factor to create your menu and put together your supplements. It's also a good year-to-year measure on your lifestyle to see if what you are currently doing is working for you.

Seven Inflammation Questions from Dr. Sears

According to Dr. Sears, if you answer yes to three of these seven questions, it's more than likely you have silent inflammation. If you do have three or more yes answers, I would recommend the stress-response diet phase one menu (more on this later).

1. Are you overweight?
2. Are you taking a statin for cholesterol?
3. Are you taking medication for elevated blood pressure?
4. Are you craving sweets or carbohydrates?
5. Are you fatigued during the day?
6. Are you groggy upon awakening in the morning?
7. Are your nails brittle?

Understanding Fats

Essential Fatty Acids (EFAs). EFAs are necessary fats that the human body needs in order to be healthy. EFAs cannot be produced by the body and must be obtained through our diet. There are two families of EFAs—omega-3 and omega-6 fatty acids. Omega-9 fatty acids are necessary, yet they are nonessential because the body can manufacture a modest amount on its own, provided the essential EFAs are present.

The human body must have EFAs to manufacture and repair cell membranes, enabling our cells to obtain optimum nutrition. EFAs are crucial in support of the cardiovascular, reproductive, immune, and nervous systems. A primary function of EFAs is the production of prostaglandins, which regulate body functions such as heart rate, blood pressure, blood clotting, fertility conception; and they play the leading role in the body's balance of its inflammation process.

As we discussed earlier, EFA deficiency and omega-6 and omega-3 imbalance has been linked with serious health conditions such as heart attacks, strokes, cancer, insulin resistance, asthma, lupus, arthritis, depression, accelerated aging, and obesity among others. It seems scientists and medical professionals are beginning to understand more and more every day about the effects of EFA imbalance and the role they play in every aspect of our health.

Omega-3 Fatty Acids (Linolenic Acid). Alpha-linolenic acid (ALA) is the principal omega-3 fatty acid, which a healthy body will convert into eicosapentaenoic acid (EPA) and, later, into docosahexaenoic acid (DHA). Omega-3 and omega-6 work together as EPA, and the gamma-linolenic acid (GLA) synthesized from omega-6 are later converted into hormone-like compounds known as eicosanoids, which aid in many bodily functions including the vital organs.

Omega-3s are essential in improving circulation and oxygen uptake for proper red blood cell function. In managing the stress response, being able to burn fat properly as our primary fuel for energy is key. This is the result of proper oxygenation in the cell, an important role of omega-3 fatty acids. Omega-3 deficiencies are linked with decreased memory, and mental abilities also associated with low oxygen levels. Omega-3 deficiencies are also associated with increased triglyceride levels, increased LDL (bad) cholesterol, hypertension, and insulin resistance among others. Look carefully and you can see these are the same diseases associated with broken down biomarkers. Bottom line, we must make sure we get an adequate amount of omega-3 fatty acids to balance the stress response and enhance every aspect of our health.

Omega-3 Foods. Omega-3 fatty acids are found in flaxseed, walnuts, pumpkin seeds, Brazil nuts, sesame seeds, avocados, salmon, mackerel, sardines, albacore tuna among others. I recommend those in the stress-response diet to supplement their diet with fish oil supplements. I recommend two to nine grams a day, depending on the client's stress levels and tested inflammation levels.

Omega-6 Fatty Acids (Linoleic Acid). Linoleic Acid (LA) is the primary omega-6 fatty acid. A healthy person with good nutrition will convert LA into GLA, which as we mentioned earlier, will be synthesized with EPA into eicosanoids. The balance of the EFAs is essential for our health management.

Most people consume too much omega-6 fatty acids in their diet. These fatty acids often are not converted to GLA because of metabolic problems (insulin resistance) caused by diets rich in sugar, alcohol, or trans fatty acids from processed foods. This conversion to GLA can also be affected by lifestyle habits such as smoking, too much stress, aging, and disease such as diabetes. It's important for our health that the omega-6 can convert to GLA so it can work with omega-3 EPA, which is essential for many bodily functions. It's best to eliminate these negative lifestyle factors when possible, but if you have many of these bad lifestyle factors, you may benefit from supplementing your diet with GLA-rich foods, such as evening primrose oil, black currant seed oil, or borage oil. Better than that, follow the stress-response diet program and the body will naturally balance itself out.

Omega-6 foods. If you are overweight or have been tested and have increased inflammation (including Dr. Sears's inflammation questions), you should keep Omega-6 foods limited in your diet and focus on increasing your omega-3s. The following foods can be consumed in small amounts: flaxseed oil, hemp seed oil, sunflower seeds, chestnut oil, corn oil, safflower oil, sunflower oil, soybean oil, and cotton seed oil—and all vegetable oil among others.

Omega-9 Fatty Acids (Oleic Acid): Omega-9 fatty acids are essential, but technically not an EFA because the human body can manufacture a limited amount. In fact, the latest research is actually showing omega-9 oleic acid can be manufactured in the liver from saturated fats (known in most circles as bad fat). More on this in "Saturated Fat."

Monounsaturated omega-9 has been shown to lower heart attack risk and arteriosclerosis and aids in lowering the affects of inflammation in the body.

Omega-9 Foods. Olive oil (extra virgin or virgin), olives, avocados, almonds, peanuts, pecans, pistachio nuts, cashews, and hazelnuts among others.

Saturated Fats: There is now a tremendous amount of research shedding new light on this so-called bad fat. The first so-called scientific proof that saturated fat was bad for us came in 1953 when a physiologist named Dr. Ancel Keys published a paper entitled "Atherosclerosis: A problem in Newer Public Health." Dr. Keys presented a comparison of fat intake and heart disease mortality in six countries—the United States, Canada, Australia, England, Italy, and Japan.

In the study, it was noted that the Americans ate the most fat and had the greatest number of deaths from heart disease; the Japanese ate the least fat and had the fewest deaths from heart disease. The other countries studied fell in-between the two. From this study came the recommendation that we continue to receive today that fat is bad. This became known as the diet-heart hypothesis. The criticism of these studies done by Dr. Keys is that many variables, that could have an impact in heart disease were left unmeasured. It was definitely true that Americans consumed more fat than the Japanese, but they also consumed more processed foods such as white bread (Wonder Bread) and were more sedentary than their Japanese counterparts. I have personally tested many clients who had high cholesterol levels and started the Atkins Diet (a very high-fat diet) to watch their cholesterol drop to normal levels after just a couple of months. These types of results fly in the face of many studies on fat and cholesterol.

The diet-heart hypothesis was and still is promoted heavily by the American Heart Association (AHA) despite new studies showing that not all saturated fat is created equal and the possibility that sugar and processed foods, not to mention our sedentary behavior, could be playing a role in the heart disease factor.

Although more than a dozen types of saturated fats exist, humans predominantly consume three:

- stearic acid
- palmitic acid
- lauric acid

This combination of saturated fats is what comprises almost 95 percent of saturated fat in a piece of steak, prime rib, slice of bacon, and nearly 70 percent of the saturated fat in butter and whole milk.

Evidence has established that stearic acid has no effect on cholesterol levels. In fact, stearic acid, which is found in high amounts in cocoa as well as animal fat such as beef and chicken, are actually converted to a monounsaturated fat oleic acid (omega-9) in the liver. This is the same heart healthy fat found in olive oil that we discussed earlier. With this evidence, scientists are now generally regarding this saturated fatty acid as either benign or potentially beneficial to your health. Maybe the late Dr. Atkins did have some validity to his concept.

The other two saturated fats, palmitic acid and lauric acid, however, are known to raise total cholesterol. But here is what is not being reported in the scientific circles—research shows that although both of these saturated fatty acids increase LDL (bad) cholesterol, they also have been shown to raise HDL (good) cholesterol just as much, if not more. And this actually lowers the risk of heart disease as we discussed earlier on the breakdown of cholesterol; it's not the overall number that matters, it's the breakdown.

This is the opposite effect that low-fat diets have on cholesterol profiles. With low-fat diets, we will have a tendency to consume more carbohydrates. When this happens, we have an increase in our triglycerides, which will lower the HDL (good) cholesterol, and thus increasing the risk of heart disease. I believe it's time for the medical field to review the research and their dietary guidelines for heart disease.

Saturated Fat
The Bottom Line

When a new client begins its evaluation process at the BioFit Center, the lipid panel (cholesterol breakdown) is one of the main tests that we order. I have personally looked at thousands of these tests over the years. When I see clients who are on low-fat diets, they end up eating too many carbohydrates while keeping the fat down in the diet. The percentage of carbohydrates is usually 60-70 percent. They will always state that they crave sweets and carbohydrates. In their profiles, they will usually have elevated triglyceride (from the carbohydrates), and this will give them a tendency to have lower than optimal HDL (good) cholesterol. The fact is that this supposedly heart-healthy menu will actually increase your risk of heart disease. When we add healthy fats to these clients menus and lower their carbohydrate intake using low-glycemic carbohydrates (more on this in the next section), we see significant changes in their profiles within as little as thirty days. The client's triglycerides drop, HDL raise, and LDL drop—all while they are consuming eggs, beef and cheese in moderation. One thing that I always say is "the testing never lies!"

The information that I have gathered over the years matches closely to what scientists are now reporting. Drs. Jeff Volek and Cassandra Forsythe from the University of Connecticut have openly questioned the public health recommendations for reducing saturated fats in the diet. They argue some saturated fats, such as stearic acid (again found in beef, chicken, and whole dairy), don't increase LDL (bad) cholesterol. One study showed that a person put on a low-fat diet containing saturated fats had a reduced progression of arterial disease. Bottom line, saturated fats don't appear to be destructive in people on a low-calorie or low-carbohydrate diet.

In the stress-response diet menu, I don't ban meat, eggs, or cheese. With that being said, *I also don't believe in micromanaged nutrition. It's not about low this or low that, it's about balance and managing the stress response.* We need to treat our diet like we would medications—with proper timing and having the right dosage (combinations of foods). Fats are important, and saturated fats should be balanced with the EFAs. Now let's take a look at the real bad fat.

Trans Fats

Trans-fatty acids are found in numerous foods—commercially packaged goods, commercially fried foods such as french fries from some fast-food chains, packaged snacks such as microwave popcorn, as well as in vegetable shortening, and some margarine. Indeed, any packaged goods that contains in its list of ingredients "partially hydrogenated vegetable oils," "hydrogenated vegetable oils," or "shortening" most likely will contain trans fats.

Trans fatty acids are manufactured fats created during a process called hydrogenation, which is a process aimed at stabilizing polyunsaturated oils to prevent them from becoming rancid (spoiled) and to keep them solid at room temperature. This allows products to stay on the shelf longer without spoiling. Hydrogenated fats are the fats used in foods such as crackers, donuts, cookies, and all processed foods that sit on the store shelf for months at a time.

Trans Fat History Lesson

When all the reports came out about how saturated fats were the cause of heart disease, the food industry immediately went to work to create an alternative fat source. The food industry wanted to switch to using unsaturated fatty acids to replace the so-called dangerous saturated fat. Unfortunately, unsaturated fatty acids spoil and become rancid rather quickly. To combat the instability of the unsaturated fatty acids, manufacturers began to hydrogenate them, a process that makes them more stable. The result was a more solid and longer-lasting form of vegetable oil called partially hydrogenated oil.

When unsaturated vegetable fats are subjected to this process of hydrogenation, a new type of fat was formed, trans fatty acids. Many manufacturers began substituting saturated fats with these new trans fatty acids, and for the first time, these fats were introduced into our mainstream diet.

The True Bad Fats

Many health professionals will tell us how bad red meat, whole dairy, and eggs are for us. The evidence out there and what I have seen over the years of conducting tests is that this just isn't true. The true bad fat would have to be the trans fat. Trans fatty acids are damaged fats that increase LDL (bad) cholesterol and actually lower the HDL (good) cholesterol, giving you a double whammy when it comes to heart disease. The irony about trans fats is that they were initially created to benefit us as an alternative to saturated fats.

Trans Fat Conclusion

In January 2006, the U.S. government took action against these fats. The government required manufacturers to list trans fat content on their nutritional labels. Manufacturers went to work to reformulate their products. Because of all the bad press about trans fats, they wanted to be able to display their products with a label that said, Zero Grams of Trans Fats. *But there is a catch. Zero grams of trans fats doesn't mean the product doesn't have these fats. The government left a loophole in the regulations that stated, "The food can still have added trans fats, but the amount has to be less than half a gram per serving."* The label can round down to zero grams as long as the manufacturer meets these guidelines. The challenge with this loophole is that the manufacturer can set the serving size to whatever it wants. In other words, a bag of chips can be several servings and state on the label that it doesn't have any trans fats. Eat a few servings of these products, which most people will do, and you have potentially eaten several grams of these bad fats.

- Trans fat exceptions. There are naturally occurring trans fatty acids that are actually healthy for the body. CLA (conjugated linoleic acid) is found in meat and whole dairy products, especially abundant in range-fed (grass-fed) cattle. A review of clinical research over the past sixteen years, published recently in the journal *Lipid Technology*, stated that CLA trans fat "has no effect or may actually lower LDL (bad) cholesterol." I have found that CLA is also a great supplement to help the body burn fat, and this is backed by many studies.
- Bio-link five: junk night. Eat deep fried foods only once a week on your day off (more on this later).

- Read the ingredient label. It's essential to read the ingredient labels closely on any packaged foods. If it says, Partially Hydrogenated Vegetable Oil or Hydrogenated Oil, try to stay away. Make sure that if the label says, zero trans fats, you read the serving size and the amount of servings per package.

Balancing fats in your diet

The main concern when it comes to balancing the fats in our diets is inflammation. We must avoid bad trans fatty acids, and we must balance our omega-6 and omega-3 fatty acids. It's essential to cut back on the omega-6 fatty acids and increase omega-3 fatty acids.

Add Omega-3

- cold-water fish like salmon, mackerel, cod, sardines, and fish oil supplements at least two grams per day.
- flaxseed
- eggs (cage free)
- walnuts
- cod liver oil
- hemp seed oil

Limit Omega-6

- most packaged foods
- canola oil
- safflower oil
- corn oil
- peanut oil
- sunflower oil
- cottonseed oil

Avoid Unhealthy Trans Fats

- fast food
- partially hydrogenated oil
- hydrogenated oil

Use Omega-9

- olives
- olive oil
- avocado
- nuts

Olive Oil

Contrary to popular belief, olive oil is a great alternative to using omega-6 oils for cooking. Olive oil has a high smoke point, 410 degrees Fahrenheit and doesn't degrade quickly as many other oils do with repeated heating.

There are many myths surrounding the use of olive oil when it comes to using this oil for cooking purposes. One myth is that olive oil will turn into a bad fat (trans fat) once it is heated. The fact is heating olive oil will not change its health aspects, only its flavor. Olive oil is a highly monounsaturated oil, and therefore, resistant to oxidation and hydrogenation, thus resistant to becoming a trans fat.

Most people wonder what is the difference between each different kind of olive oil. Should I use extra virgin, virgin, or plain olive oil? The difference between the oils is their acidity level, which affects the taste, not the nutritional content of the oil. The lower acidity of the oil, such as extra virgin, tends to have more antioxidants. I tend to recommend pure or plain olive oil for cooking and extra virgin olive oil for salads and foods. Remember that olive oil is an omega-9 fatty acid and does not contain the EFAs. It's a great oil to have in the house, especially for food preparation and flavor, but we must still stay focused on the omega-6/omega-3 inflammation equation.

Weight-Loss Fat?

Before closing this section on fat, I would like to share a secret fat that can actually help us lose weight. We talked earlier about the many misconceptions of saturated fats. We do have to keep our saturated fat intake under control, but we do not have to avoid them. One saturated fat that we have been taught over the years to be bad for our health is coconut oil. This couldn't be further from the truth, in fact, this may be a fat that burns fat. When we take a look at coconut oil, it is 92 percent saturated fat and has been on every food avoid list for the last thirty years. How could this oil ever be considered healthy?

Coconut may be high in saturated fat, but it is also a high source of what is called a medium-chain triglyceride (MCTs), and MCTs have been shown to actually raise the body's metabolism because the body directly uses MCTs for energy. Coconut-derived MCTs increase fat burning and thermogenic effects up to 50 percent. This is due to the coconut oil's absorbability, which reduces the strain on the pancreas (decreased insulin) and digestive system. For this reason, coconut helps regulate blood sugar by minimizing insulin spikes.

Reasons to Consider Coconut

- Coconuts and coconut oil are a great alternative for cooking and flavoring foods because they are supportive of general health, contrary to popular belief.
- Coconut oil is also an antiviral; it actually attacks and kills many viruses.
- Coconut acts more like a carbohydrate than a fat. It is great for weight loss because it is used quickly for energy, so it is not stored like other fats.
- Coconut oil has been shown to support thyroid function.
- Coconut oil improves the body's use of blood glucose and improves insulin secretion and absorption.
- Coconut oil improves digestion and absorption of fat-soluble vitamins, minerals, and amino acids.
- Coconut oil is a natural antioxidant and protects the body from free radicals.

Carbohydrates

Carbohydrates are one of the most important foods to understand and to control for the stress-response diet. Carbohydrates are the main source of blood glucose, which is a major fuel for all our cells, and as we mentioned previously, the only source of fuel for our brain and nervous system. Carbohydrates are found almost exclusively in plant foods, such as fruit, vegetables, grains, and beans. Milk is probably the only animal-derived food that has carbohydrates.

Most of us have been taught that carbohydrates are divided into two groups—simple and complex carbohydrates. Simple carbohydrates are also known as simple sugars. Among these, we include fruit (fructose), table sugar (sucrose), and milk (lactose). These are the three main sugars. Complex carbohydrates are also made up of sugars, but the sugar molecules are strung together to form longer and more complex chains. Complex carbohydrates include vegetables, whole grains, peas, beans, and legumes.

In the last thirty years, the recommendation of the medical community has been to cut the fat out of your diet for health and weight loss. This information makes complete sense when we examine the facts—fat has nine calories per gram while proteins and carbohydrates only have four calories per gram. Simply put, cut the fat, cut the calories, and we will lose weight. This simple solution to weight loss led to an explosion in new marketing and new foods called reduced fat and fat free. However, with time, the low-fat recommendations didn't translate into positive results; in fact, quite the opposite happened. In the last two decades, the obesity rate in the United States has risen from 46 percent to 56 percent.

Let's be honest, we cannot just blame the low-fat movement with the rise of obesity, there are larger portions, more junk food and sedentary lifestyles that are also to blame. But it cannot be denied with what we know today that the low-fat diet movement had a lot to do with it. The facts are simple; the reduction of fats in foods has been accomplished by increasing the level of refined carbohydrates (sugars) in their content. These carbohydrates are broken down too quickly into glucose by the digestive system for the body to be able to immediately make use of them. As we have learned, this will cause a spike in blood glucose levels, causing a spike in insulin to get the sugar out of the bloodstream. The cells are filled with glucose while the excess sugar is the converted into fat. These foods high in refined sugars completely throw off the stress response, causing a fast rise of insulin and then a quick drop, leaving the body in a hypoglycemic condition (low blood sugar). When this happens, we have cravings, extreme hunger, and we cannot burn fat. Bottom line, we are completely out of balance. This imbalance causes the body to store fat and crave sweets and in time, will cause us to become insulin resistant and develop such diseases such as metabolic syndrome and diabetes. The high-carbohydrate diet has not and cannot work. Fats, on the other hand, while containing more calories per gram, are more slowly digested and produce a feeling of satiety for a longer period of time. The average fatty meal takes four to six hours to digest, raising the metabolism in the process. When our diet has the proper fats, we will actually eat less calories throughout the day, thus we lose weight.

Good versus Bad Carbohydrates

We must have carbohydrates as part of our diet. We have discussed in the cycles of health that as we age, most of us will have more problems processing carbohydrates. That doesn't mean we must remove them from our diet. The popular no-carbohydrate approaches, which advocate a no-carbohydrate intake is not the answer to permanent health and fat loss either. It's also not the answer to balancing the stress response. No-carbohydrate diets introduce a rather simple philosophy. Basically, the body has two fuel sources—carbohydrates and fats. If you want the body to burn fat, then remove the carbohydrates.

The no-carbohydrate approach is right in theory, but in practice, it is missing something. It is true, the body has two fuel sources, but as we discussed earlier, the brain has only one fuel source—sugar broken down from carbohydrates. If we don't have a balanced menu for our particular metabolism, the body will then break down the muscle and the biomarkers. When the biomarkers break down, we accelerate aging, destroy our metabolism, and stop burning fat for energy.

The key is not to remove carbohydrates from your diet but to take in the right type of carbohydrates with the right combinations of food and at the right time of the day. This is key for us to manage the stress response, as one of the most important hormones we must manage for our health and any type of fat burning is insulin. Every time we eat carbohydrates, they are broken down into sugar (again all carbs are broken down into sugar), and the body releases insulin to get the sugar out of the bloodstream. This response determines if a carbohydrate is good or bad. One of the keys to burning fat is eating the carbohydrates that minimize the insulin release. The slower the carbohydrate breaks down, the less insulin is released. I call this insulin management.

Insulin Management

High insulin is the common enemy of most dieters as we discussed in the section "The Ten Reasons the Body Stops Burning Fat." The number one reason is insulin resistance. Insulin is critical for glucose metabolism, storage, and maintenance. Insulin wasn't meant to be released in excessive levels as it is when a person is on a low-fat, high-carbohydrate diet or when they consume refined carbohydrates. When food is consumed, the digestive process converts carbohydrates into glucose, a simple sugar, which is absorbed into the bloodstream. The pancreas releases insulin in response to blood glucose. Insulin then enters certain cells and triggers events that cause the cell to absorb glucose from the blood (explained in chapter 9 in detail). The consumption of excessive amounts of refined carbohydrates or a change in the way the body metabolizes carbohydrates (cycles of health) can result in insulin resistance, the loss of sensitivity to insulin by many tissue cells. The body responds by producing even more insulin, which results in elevated insulin and glucose levels, which shuts down any chances of the body-burning fat (chapter nine for more details on insulin resistance and fat burning).

Managing insulin is about taking in the right type of carbohydrates and not all carbohydrates are created equal. Certain carbohydrates lead the body to release glucose faster into the blood than it can be used by the body, that is the problem—those with a high glycemic index (GI) in particular have this characteristic. These high-glycemic foods are what cause an imbalance when it comes to managing insulin.

The Glycemic Index

The glycemic index measures the glycemia of a food (how fast it breaks down into sugar) and it was first developed in 1981. The concept is that the higher the blood sugar level, the more insulin the body has to release. The lower the glycemic number, the slower the food breaks down into sugar. The more stable the blood sugar level remains, the less insulin is released. This is the key to insulin management.

The glycemic index rates foods from zero to one hundred, with one hundred being pure glucose. Before the development of the glycemic index in 1981, scientists assumed that our bodies absorbed and digested simple sugars quickly, producing a rapid increase in our blood sugar levels. Now we know that simple sugars do not necessarily make your blood sugar rise any more rapidly than some complex carbohydrates. The determining factor is the glycemic index and how fast the sugar breaks down in the body.

High-Glycemic Carbohydrates

The best way to picture how high-glycemic carbohydrates break down in the body is to imagine a glass sitting in a sink under the water faucet. Imagine you open the faucet at full capacity all of a sudden. The glass will fill up in seconds, and water will begin to spill out of the glass quickly. This is the same way sugar floods into your body, causing what is called an insulin spike, because the body overproduces insulin to rid the body of sugar. This is bad insulin management.

We talked about the fact that fat doesn't make us fat. It's high GI carbohydrates that are the main culprit. Let's take a look at the process one more time. It is so important to understand. We eat the high GI carbohydrate; the body turns them immediately into (glucose) sugar. The final destination of glucose is to be stored as glycogen in the muscle cell. The muscle is like a sponge; when the muscle cells are full of glycogen, they close their doors. This leaves excess sugar in the bloodstream, causing more insulin to be released. This insulin then takes the sugar to the liver where triglycerides (blood fat) and cholesterol are produced. The liver, with the help of VLDL (very low-density lipoprotein) takes the excess fat and stores it somewhere in the body.

Low-Glycemic Carbohydrates

Low-glycemic carbohydrates enter the body slowly. Picture the glass below the water faucet, only this time, the water drips slowly into the glass. This prevents a spike and keeps a healthy blood sugar level. The body releases insulin in amounts proportionate to the sugar levels, and it easily stores the sugar away. Once the sugar is stored, insulin shuts down and then frees the body to release glucagon so fat burning can begin. Low-glycemic carbohydrates help us to manage our insulin levels. When you consume low-glycemic carbohydrates along with the right combinations of fats and proteins, you manage the stress response. When you manage the stress response, you manage the insulin levels. With low-glycemic carbohydrates, you do not get cravings for sweets, sudden energy crashes, or hormonal imbalances as you do with high-glycemic carbohydrates.

Low-Glycemic Load

The fact is our body needs carbohydrates in order to maintain a healthy balance. Another fact is that as we get older and travel through the cycles of health, our bodies will have more trouble with processing these carbohydrates. Many low-carbohydrate advocates just make all carbohydrates out as evil. This point of view is an oversimplification; just as stating all fats are bad (as we have learned this is not true). It's about how much and how fast the sepcific carbohydrate releases glucose into the blood. Those with the higher glycemic index tend to have this negative effect. While the glycemic index itself is important as a measurement of how quickly and how high blood glucose levels may rise per each particular food, it is important to keep in mind that eating large amounts of moderate glycemic index foods can lead to blood glucose levels that are too high. In other words, the portion and the amount of the food can make a difference. A useful concept I have been using in the last couple of years is the glycemic load (GL).

The glycemic load is a relatively new way to assess the impact of carbohydrate consumption. The glycemic load takes the glycemic index into account but gives a clearer picture than the glycemic index alone. A glycemic index value tells you only how rapidly a particular carbohydrate turns into sugar. It doesn't tell you how much of that carbohydrate is in a serving of a particular food. The glycemic load on the other hand gives us a more complete picture. An example of a food that for years was on the stress-response diet avoid list was watermelon. Watermelon has a high glycemic index value of seventy-two (GI value above fifty-five is considered high). But the overall carbohydrate content of watermelon is low, so the glycemic load is four (GL value below ten is considered low). Watermelon will not cause a glucose overload or an insulin spike. More on this in the next chapter.

Measuring the Glycemic Load

The glycemic load uses the amount of carbohydrates and the glycemic index of a particular food to give us more of a complete breakdown of the carbohydrate. To calculate the GL in a typical serving of food, divide the GI of that food by one hundred and multiply the result by the amount of carbohydrates per serving of the particular food. For example, the glycemic index of carrots is around 47. Carrots contain about 7 grams of carbohydrates per 100 g of carrots. To calculate the glycemic load for a standard 50-g serving of carrots, divide 47 by 100 (0.47) and multiply by 3.5. The glycemic load of carrots is therefore 1.6.

(glycemic index value) x (amount of carbs per serving) divided by 100 = GL

GI of 70 or more   High
GI of 56 to 69   Medium
GI of 55 or less   Low

GL of 20 or more   High
GL of 11 to 19   Medium
GL of 10 or less   Low

Using the glycemic load can make a much more accurate menu. Let me give you an example of two foods—spaghetti and apples. Both these foods have a glycemic index of forty.

Spaghetti.

GI: 40. One cup serving has 52 grams of carbohydrates.
$$\text{Glycemic Load} = (40 \times 52) / 100$$
$$= 20.8 \text{ (High)}$$

Apple.

GI: 40. One medium apple has 15 grams of carbohydrates.
$$\text{Glycemic Load} = (40 \times 15) / 100$$
$$= 6 \text{ (Low)}$$

As you can see from the examples above, there is a significant difference in the two foods glycemic loads even though they have the same glycemic index value. The stress-response diet is designed to create a low-glycemic load with its food combinations and menu phases. We will discuss this further when we build your menu.

Glycemic index values 55 or below are considered low, and values 70 or above are considered high. Glycemic load values of 10 or below are considered low, and values 20 or above are considered high. Because the glycemic index is so extent I couldn't include it in its entirety in this book but, I recommend the official Website of the glycemic index and glycemic load database as a reference, ***www.glycemicindex.com.*** In this website you can research all the foods you like and use it to put together the lists of foods that will make up your menu.

• Food	• GI	• Serving Size	• Net Carbs	• GL
• Peanuts	• 14	• 4oz (113g)	• 15	• 2
• Bean Sprouts	• 25	• 1 cup (104g)	• 4	• 1
• Grapefruit	• 25	• ½ lg (1669g)	• 11	• 3
• Pizza	• 30	• 2 sl (2609g)	• 42	• 13
• Low Fat Yogurt	• 33	• 1 cup (245g)	• 47	• 16
• Apples	• 38	• 1 Med (131g)	• 16	• 6
• Spaghetti	• 40	• 1 Cup (140g)	• 52	• 20
• Carrots	• 47	• 1 lg (72g)	• 5	• 2
• Orange	• 48	• 1 Med (131g)	• 12	• 6
• Brown Rice	• 50	• ¾ cup (150g)	• 50	• 16
• Banana	• 52	• 1 lg (136g)	• 27	• 14
• Wheat Bread	• 53	• 1 slice (30g)	• 53	• 11
• Potato Chips	• 54	• 4oz (114g)	• 55	• 30
• Snickers Bar	• 55	• 1 bar (113g)	• 64	• 35
• Honey	• 55	• 1 tbsp (21g)	• 17	• 9
• Oatmeal	• 58	• 1 serv (234g)	• 21	• 12
• Sweet Potato	• 61	• 1 med (150g)	• 30	• 18
• Ice Cream	• 61	• 1 cup (72g)	• 16	• 10
• Macaroni/Cheese	• 64	• 1 serv (166g)	• 47	• 30
• Raisins	• 64	• 1 sm box (43g)	• 32	• 20
• White Rice	• 64	• 1 cup (186g)	• 52	• 33
• Sugar (sucrose)	• 66	• 1 Tbsp (12g)	• 12	• 8
• White Bread	• 70	• 1 slice (30g)	• 14	• 10
• Watermelon	• 72	• 1 cup (154g)	• 11	• 8
• Popcorn	• 72	• 2 cups (169g)	• 10	• 7
• Baked Potato	• 85	• 1 med (173g)	• 33	• 28
• Glucose	• 100	• (50g)	• 50	• 50

Table 2

The glycemic index and the glycemic load are key tools in the stress-response diet. Rapid increases in blood sugar following a high glycemic index meal triggers greater insulin release, which speeds sugar transport into cells and promotes fat storage. This effect from high-glycemic carbohydrates also has an effect on the stress-response hormones cortisol and insulin. I have found that carbohydrate foods are the one category of food that has to be individually controlled to create a balanced menu.

Calories

What about the calories in the diet? During my diet years of losing and gaining weight, I was always told that a calorie is a calorie. If you want to lose weight, the formula is simple: eat less, exercise more. This seems to be a common-sense approach; the only problem is that it doesn't work. Anyone who has ever been on the weight-loss roller coaster (especially after age thirty-five) will tell you that this formula is doomed to fail. Even if you do lose weight, you will always gain it back. Many of the overweight clients that I see don't really eat that much. If you really analyze their total calories and their basal metabolic rate (BMR), you would be surprised that many don't consume that many calories over their BMR. They usually only eat one to two times a day and consume a lot of their calories in a couple of meals. But looking at the formula that a calorie is a calorie, they shouldn't be obese. It's what and when they eat that throws the body into a state of imbalance. Basically, the truth is it's the chemistry of the individual's diet that really matters. You must eat the right combinations of food at the right times throughout the day so you can balance the stress response. Without balancing the stress-response hormones, the body cannot possibly burn fat. One of the hormones that get out of balance when the stress response is off is leptin. Leptin is crucial for our body to be able to lose weight (fat).

We talked about leptin earlier when we discussed the fat-burning hormones. It is important to revisit this hormone, especially when discussing calories. The medical community in general embeds the calorie myth theory. The whole premise of the stress-response diet is that we have inborn, natural regulatory systems that support a healthy weight. These systems are part of our survival mechanism and it's coded into our survival DNA. Unfortunately, this mechanism is designed for us to survive in a cave. Our lifestyle choices, the foods that we consume, and our daily activity levels have a direct relation on the survival mechanism and the stress response. Leptin is one of the key hormones for any type of weight loss (fat) to take place. Leptin is a compound that lets your brain and body know how much fat you are storing. When leptin levels rise, your appetite will go down. Leptin also speeds up your metabolism and signals the body to either burn or store fat. The problem with overweight people is that they have developed leptin resistance. Leptin resistance is when their leptin levels are high (which is good), but it is not connecting to the brain. In other words, without the brain connection, the body perceives that leptin levels are actually low. So the leptin is not suppressing their appetites, not stimulating their metabolism, and they cannot burn fat no matter how little their calorie intakes may be.

Losing Weight
Sandra's Story

Sandra is a forty-five-year-old mother of three. Sandra is an executive secretary to a top CEO of a large company. When I met Sandra, she had just had gastric bypass surgery. She was feeling extremely tired and was having trouble with her meals and taking in any type of solid foods. Sandra had a history of obesity and had been dieting most of her adult life. Sandra weighed 378 pounds and had a body composition of 43.4 percent body fat. The doctor that sent Sandra to me had set specific goals for her. One of the goals was she could not start an exercise program until she was down to 300 pounds. We worked closely on Sandra's diet, helping her to work in more solid food and prevent any digestion problems. After eight weeks, Sandra lost fifty pounds. The doctor was very enthusiastic, but I explained to him that this actually wasn't good. When we did Sandra's body composition, her body fat was still 43.2 percent. The doctor still rejected the possibility of her starting an exercise program. Within another thirty days, she lost another twenty-two pounds. She was feeling weak and very tired. When we did her body composition assessment, her body fat was exactly where she started at 43.4 percent even though she had lost over seventy pounds. Then, the doctor let us start her on an exercise program. In the next six months, she lost an additional seventy-two pounds, but this time, her body fat percentage dropped to 26 percent. Not only did Sandra look great for the first time in years, she also felt great with an abundance of energy and strength she hadn't had since she was a teenager.

Many people are like Sandra and her doctor when it comes to weight loss; the more the scale drops, the better. This just isn't true when it comes to overall health and age management. If you are losing muscle, you are breaking down the biomarkers and that will result in weight regained plus less muscle and metabolism. Sandra was eating very few calories, but her body's stress response was out of balance, causing her body to go into a survival state and preserve its fat stores at all costs.

Diet Chemistry and Combination Is
More Important than Calories

Everything that we have discussed throughout this book has one theme, and that is balance. It is not always about calories; what is most important about your food intake is how it affects the chemistry of your body. That is the key that will result in permanent weight (fat) loss and good health.

Health is achieved by balancing the stress response and that becomes more increasingly difficult after age thirty-five. Our diet plays a crucial role in keeping the stress response balanced and keeping the leptin hormone communications clear. When it comes to diet, the old adage "a little cannot hurt" does not apply after we enter the second cycle of health. If you take a bite of a chocolate cake, for example, it has an effect on your insulin response that will throw the other hormones out of balance. This will cause you to crave more cake. It's important to follow your menu for six days, and then take a day off. We will discuss this more in bio-link five.

The combinations of food also play a strong role in balancing the stress response. One of the first things students learn in nutrition 101 is all calories are the same. However, several well-controlled studies show people lose more weight on low-carbohydrate diets than they do on mixed or high-carbohydrate diets. Some researchers think that the high protein diets require more calories to metabolize while others feel protein cuts appetite. The truth is that when you add protein throughout the day, you balance the stress response. When the body has the stress response balanced, you will not crave or be overly hungry, and then your body will burn fat for energy. The combinations and timing of our meals are essential in creating a thermogenic effect. When we are balanced, we have no real need to count calories because the body simply will not want to overeat.

Chapter Sixteen

Constructing Your Stress-Response Diet

Health is a state of complete physical, mental and social wellbeing, and not merely the absence of disease or infirmity.
—*World Health Organization, 1948*

The stress-response diet menu is about the proper combinations of foods that we need in order to balance the stress response. Each food group is important to achieve balance and fat burning.

- Carbohydrates control insulin which is a hormone directly related to the stress response. Carbohydrates are essential for brain function but, also need to be low glycemic and properly timed. Vegetables, grains, beans, fruit all fall in this category.
- Proteins are essential for the body's ability to repair itself. Recuperation is the key to balancing the stress response in today's fast-paced world.
- Healthy fat intake is the key to controlling silent inflammation. This is essential for our body's ability to burn fat and determines our long-term health.
- When setting up your plate during Phase I keep in mind to divide it this way: One quarter of the plate must have a protein food and the rest of the plate must have vegetables. These vegetables can be salads, broccoli, cauliflower and other vegetables.
- When setting up your plate during Phase II and Phase III one quarter of the plate will have your protein, one quarter will have a serving of whole grains such as brown rice, whole wheat pasta or sweet potato.

The other half of the plate must be made up of vegetables and salads. The reason for this breakdown is to maintain the proper alkaline balance in the body.

The other key element for the stress-response diet menu to be effective is the timing of the meals. Snacks are very important to balance the stress response. We will discuss what types of snacks later, but first, let's take a look at the phases of the menus.

Promoting Metabolic Health

During prehistoric times, cavemen lived on vegetables, fruits, meats, beans, and roots. Our genes haven't changed over the last ten thousand years all that much, but our diet, physical activity levels, and the daily amount of stress we are under have. As we have discussed, our stress response is programmed for survival during prehistoric times, and we are genetically programmed to thrive on the caveman diet. Our modern processed-food diet works against the stress response because it imbalances the hormones, which can promote cardiovascular disease, diabetes, and cancer. A group of Swedish researchers showed that pigs consuming the caveman-type diet were leaner and showed better blood sugar control and lower diastolic blood pressure. They also showed lower levels of inflammation than pigs that were fed a cereal-based diet. Scientist study pigs because they develop coronary artery disease and diabetes similar to humans. Today's modern diet shows that we are taking in more calories, saturated and trans fats, cereal grains and take in fewer omega-3 fats, fiber, fruits and vegetables, protein, and calcium. The stress response is directly affected by the modern diet. The stress-response diet is designed to give the body what it needs to create proper energy and maintain stress balance.

Three Menu Phases

Phase one menu. This menu is designed to cleanse the body and balance the stress response. Phase one is more limited on carbohydrates, and this allows us to manage the insulin response, which in turn balances the stress response. Phase one doesn't usually become the permanent lifestyle menu, but for some like myself who don't process carbohydrates well, this is the menu I live with six days a week. You will know if this is the right phase for you because you will experience high energy levels, no cravings for sweets, and will not be starving at night.

Phase one guidelines:

- Follow phase one for thirty days and then reevaluate whether to move to phase two. If you are experiencing cravings for carbohydrates (when following the program), headaches, and fatigue, go to phase two, but only after thirty days. If you feel energetic and experience no cravings, you can safely remain on phase one until you are ready.
- Phase one is a cleansing phase menu. It is designed to help your body balance the stress response by balancing sugar and insulin. Be patient. It takes one to two weeks to cleanse the body, and you will begin to feel great.
- Phase one menu is split into five meals—three main meals and two snacks.
- Low-glycemic fruit is allowed at breakfast only, *no juices are allowed.*
- The morning snack can be either protein or fats (check the snack options).
- The afternoon snack between lunch and dinner needs to be protein, preferably a whey protein supplement.
- Grains are only allowed at breakfast.
- Healthy fats must be included in all three main meals.
- When preparing your food in phase one, you can use olive oil or Pam Spray for cooking. You can use spices, herbs, lime or lemon juice, and pepper and mustard as condiments. You can also add low-fat white cheese to your protein and vegetables to enliven the flavor of your foods if you choose to. Be creative with your meals, but stay true to the ingredients suggested.
- Most restaurants will easily conform to the stress-response diet menu. You must ask for what you want and avoid the foods that you are not allowed. Instead of the bread appetizers, order vegetables, soups, or salad such as a caprece salad. This menu is easy to follow.
- The soups recommended in phase one should be low sodium and without a cream base. They should be a broth type or vegetables base, and not have any starches included.
- Yogurts should be no-sugar-added or plain. (But you may add Stevia, truvia or Splenda to sweeten them).

Phase one menu example:

Breakfast
- Protein: Omelet with one whole egg and two egg whites with an ounce of white cheese.
- Grains: ½ cup natural oatmeal (make sure it has no sugar added).
- Vegetables: Onions and mushrooms in the omelet; *unlimited* low-glycemic vegetables; no starchy vegetables.
- Fruit: Three to five ounces of fresh berries (put into the oatmeal).
- Fats: Cook the omelet in one teaspoon of olive oil or use ten almonds to mix into the oatmeal. Another option is to add flaxseed to the meal.

Morning snack (three hours after breakfast)
- Twelve to twenty-four whole almonds

Lunch (three hours after AM snack)
- Protein: Three to six ounces of grilled chicken breast with spices, lemon, herbs, vinegar, or mustard for flavor. (You can replace the chicken with meat or fish if you would like).
- Grains: Three and a half ounces of lentils
- Vegetables: Unlimited low-glycemic vegetables; no starchy vegetables; tossed salad with oil/vinegar dressing.
- Fruit: None
- Fats: Two teaspoons to one tablespoon of olive oil.
- One ounce of sugar-free dark chocolate (70 percent cocoa or higher).

Afternoon Snack (three hours after lunch)
- Whey protein drink with twenty to thirty grams of protein.

Dinner (three hours after PM Snack)
- Protein: Three to six ounces of grilled fillet steak (lean cut) or chicken or fish.
- Grains: None
- Vegetables: Unlimited low-glycemic vegetables; no starchy vegetables; salad with light dressing on the side (low sugar).
- Fruits: None
- Fats: Olives in the salad or olive oil or both.
- Sugar-free Jell-O

Phase Two Menu. This menu can be used for a lifetime of wellness. Phase two allows more carbohydrates throughout the day, but still limits them at night to maximize the stress response. Very few of us need carbohydrates at night as we don't need to use our brains when we are asleep. Also, many times, too many carbohydrates at night will tend to throw the stress response out of balance. Phase two is a great fat-burning menu.

Phase two guidelines:

- Follow the phase two menu from thirty to sixty days for maximum benefit. As I mentioned above, you can remain on this menu forever. You can also stay on the phase two menu until you reach your goals, and then proceed to phase three.
- Phase two is a great fat-burning menu as it controls insulin at night, which allows the body to easily burn fat while you sleep. (Obviously, phase one does the same).
- Phase two menu is split into five meals—three main meals and two snacks.
- Low to medium-glycemic fruit is allowed at breakfast, morning snack (*fruit must be eaten with a healthy fat or protein, never by itself, as it will throw off the stress response*) and lunch.
- The afternoon snack between lunch and dinner needs to be protein, preferably a whey protein supplement.
- Grains are allowed at breakfast, morning snack—combined with a protein or fat—and lunch. Try to make the grains low-medium glycemic.
- When preparing your food in phase two, you can use olive oil, Pam Spray, or a small amount of butter for cooking. You can use spices, herbs, lime or lemon juice, and pepper and mustard as condiments. You can also add low-fat white cheese to your protein and vegetables to enliven the flavor of your foods if you choose. Be creative with your meals, but stay true to the ingredients suggested.
- Most restaurants will easily conform to the stress-response diet menu. When eating out, you know what you cannot have. Ask for soups as an appetizer or raw vegetables. Salads, such as a caprice salad, are great starters. This program is very easy because you will not crave carbohydrates. If you cannot get healthy carbohydrates, it is better to skip the carbohydrate than throw off your stress response. Remember, grains and legumes are also grains.
- The soups recommended should not be cream-based and without starch-based vegetables.

- Avoid white rice, potato, white bread, and white pasta that are overcooked. Al dente pasta in small amounts is fine (better if you mix olive oil with it).
- Yogurts should be no sugar added or plain.

Phase Two Menu Example:

Breakfast
- Protein: a half cup of cottage cheese
- Grains: One to two slices of whole grain bread with sugar-free jelly (you can replace the toast with half a cup of natural oatmeal with no sugar added).
- Vegetables: sliced tomato
- Fruits: Small glass of sugar-free, natural orange juice with pulp or some pineapple to mix with the cottage cheese.
- Fats: Eight to twelve whole almonds (mix into the cottage cheese)

AM Snack
- Whole-grain crackers with some natural peanut butter or sugar-free yogurt with fruit.

Lunch
- Protein: Three and a half to six ounces of grilled salmon with herbs, spices, and some lemon. (You can replace the salmon with meat or chicken).
- Grains: Three to four ounces or a half cup of wild rice with a half cup of lentils.
- Vegetables: Unlimited low-glycemic vegetables; soup of chicken broth; and vegetables.
- Fruits: Dessert of mixed berries
- Fats: 1 tablespoon olive oil over vegetable

PM Snack
- Whey protein supplement twenty to thirty grams mixed with strawberries or sugar-free yogurt with whey protein mixed in.

Dinner
- Protein: Three to six ounces of lean beef (fillet, trim off excess fat). You can replace the beef with chicken or fish.

- Grains: None
- Vegetables: Unlimited low-glycemic vegetables; mixed salad with salad leaves, tomato, cucumber, red onion, radish, and one teaspoon olive oil/vinegar dressing. Eat hearty.
- Fruits: none
- Fats: One teaspoon of olive oil
- Misc: Dark chocolate for dessert two to four ounces or a glass of red wine

Phase three menu. This is the maintenance menu phase and is a guideline for the way you will be eating to maintain your results and a lifetime of wellness. Phase three will balance the stress response and give you not only permanent fat loss, but also great energy levels and healthy longevity. Phase three should only be used once you have reached your goals from phase two.

Phase three guidelines:

- Phase three is followed as your daily menu to balance the stress response. This is the menu you will use for a lifetime. If you start to experience fatigue, cravings for carbohydrate, or weight gain while using this phase, it simply means you are a phase-two person and need to use that menu for maintenance.
- Phase three menu is split into five meals—three main meals and two snacks.
- Low-glycemic fruit is allowed in all the meals and snacks, except at the dinner meal. It's still good to keep sugar a minimum at night to keep the stress response balanced. Sugar's main function is to fuel the brain, and we don't need our brain functioning when we sleep. The same rules apply with fruit here; never eat fruit alone in the snacks, always with a protein or a fat.
- It is recommended, if you have a lifestyle of high stress, to make the afternoon snack between lunch and dinner a whey protein snack. This snack must be protein but can be mixed with low-glycemic carbohydrates.
- Grains are allowed throughout the day. They must be low-medium glycemic.
- When preparing your foods in phase three, you can use olive oil or Pam Spray or a small amount of butter for cooking. You can

use spices, herbs, lime or lemon juice, and pepper and mustard as
condiments. You can also add low-fat white cheese to your protein
and vegetables to enliven the flavor of your foods if you choose
to. Be creative with your meals, but stay true to the ingredients
suggested.

- Most restaurants will easily conform to the stress-response diet menu.
  When eating out, you must avoid white rice, white potato, white
  bread, and white pasta that is overcooked (al dente is fine). When
  you cannot get the healthy grains, skip them; it's better not to eat
  the carbohydrates than throw off the stress response. Remember,
  beans and legumes are also grains.
- Yogurts should be no sugar added or plain.

Phase three menu example:

Breakfast
- Protein: Twenty to thirty grams whey protein mixed into the
  oatmeal.
- Grains: Half a cup of natural oatmeal with no sugar added. You can
  replace the oatmeal with two whole wheat or whole grain slices of
  bread.
- Vegetables: None
- Fruits: A half cup of strawberries mixed into the oatmeal.
- Fats: Twelve whole almonds mixed into the oatmeal.

AM Snack
- Three ounces of cottage cheese mixed with pineapple.

Lunch
- Protein: Three to seven ounces of chicken breast (with herbs and
  seasoning). You can replace the chicken with meat or fish.
- Grains: A cup of whole-grain pasta with tomato sauce and seasonings.
  You can replace the pasta with brown rice or two slices of whole
  wheat or whole grain bread.
- Vegetables: unlimited low-glycemic vegetables
- Fruit: Half a cup of mixed fruit for dessert.
- Fats: One tablespoon of olive oil for the vegetables and chicken

PM Snack
- Twenty grams whey protein mixed with fruit and yogurt.

Dinner
- Protein: Omelet made from two whole eggs and two whites with mixed vegetables and an ounce of mozzarella cheese. You can replace the omelet with meat, chicken, or fish.
- Grains: Two slices of rye bread with a pat of butter.
- Vegetables: Half a cup of low-glycemic vegetables mixed with the omelet.
- Fruits: none
- Fats: One teaspoon of olive oil, used in preparing the omelet.
- Misc. One cup of no-sugar-added ice cream for dessert.

Choosing Your Menu Phase

When clients come into the BioFit Centers, I do not guess which phase menu they need. At the Center, we use advanced testing to determine the right phase of each menu. We use an electro lipo graphic (ELG) test to measure the clients' biomarkers and body composition. We also run specific blood tests according to the client's history and the cardio-metabolic stress test (bio-energy) results. With this information, we take out the guesswork from the client's lifestyle programs. Over the years and after seeing many clients, I have identified ten markers you can use to find out which is the right phase menu for you. These are the ten markers, simply answer yes or no:

1. Do you fell overweight? (If you weight more than you did last year or your clothes fit tighter, or if you changed clothes sizes, mark yes)
2. Do you have a family history of heart disease?
3. Do you have a family history of diabetes?
4. Do you have insulin resistance? When it comes to insulin resistance, it's not how much fat you have that is important; it's where you store it. Researchers from the Washington University School of Medicine in St. Louis found that abdominal adiposity, as measured by waist circumference, was a better predictor of insulin resistance than aerobic capacity (BMI or percent of fat). If you store most of

your fat around the waist, mark yes. If you have been diagnosed by a Doctor with insulin resistance, mark yes.

5. Are your stress levels seven or higher on a scale of one to ten? I know they go up and down, but where would you put an average?
6. Do you experience cravings for sweets or carbohydrates?
7. Energy. Over the last six months, on a scale of one to ten, where would you rate you energy levels? Below seven, mark yes.
8. Inflammation. Do you experience joint pain and have more frequent illnesses?
9. Do you have trouble sleeping or you wake up in the middle of the night and cannot get back to sleep?
10. Are you in the third cycle of health (forty-five to fifty-five years)? Most people gain weight as they age, particularly in the abdomen. This is mainly due to the body's ability to process carbohydrates. A diet that was perfect at forty years of age may no longer work at forty-five.

Phase one menu. If you answered five or more questions with a yes, start with phase one. Stay on phase one for at least the first thirty days, and then reassess yourself and go to phase two. If you find that you are really feeling great, then stay with it. If you start feeling tired, having cravings for sweets, and headaches, move on to phase two.

Phase two menu. If you answered three to four questions with a yes, start on phase two for at least thirty to sixty days. You can safely remain on this phase until you reach your goals.

Phase three menu. If you answered two or fewer questions with a yes, you can easily get results on the phase three menu.

Creating Your Tailored Menu

Here is a basic list of good and bad foods that I would like for you to follow. Go to your phase sample and simply plug in your food choices for the phase menu you are on. Here, you will also find easy tips for portion control and metabolic eating to boost your metabolism and easily manage calories without counting. For a more complete list of exchange foods per phase, visit the web site at www.biofitprogram.com.

What-to-avoid list for all phases:

Proteins to Limit

For the most part, there is no need to avoid protein foods. It's the fatty proteins that you have to keep limited, especially if you suffer from elevated cholesterol.

- Bacon. This should be limited to once a week and no more than two to three pieces.
- Fatty Beef. Always choose the leaner cuts of beef.
- Liver. This includes chicken and lamb liver. Actually, liver can be a very nutritious source of protein. The reason you should limit the amount is because the liver is a detoxifying organ of the body, so that means it is quite likely to contain toxins. If you do eat liver, try to consume calf's liver as it is from the younger animal and may be a little healthier.
- Salami. It's all right to have small amounts of salami as a treat, but it should not be a regular part of your menu.
- Hot Dog. I really don't have to say too much here. Again, like salami, you can have a hot dog as a treat once a week either at a ball game or at a bar-B-Q if you want..

Grains to Limit

To manage the stress response, we must manage the body's insulin levels; therefore, you must limit the following foods to once a week (you may have some only on junk day).

- White bread. This includes everything from bagels to pita to crackers
- White rice. This includes rice cakes
- White potato. This includes baked, boiled, and fried ones (starchy vegetable)
- White pasta. Only when overcooked. Pasta al dente is lower glycemic, but portions must be managed.
- Potato chips. This includes all types of corn chips.
- Pastries. This includes things like doughnuts, cookies, etc.
- Cereals. It's important to check the GL of your favorite cereals. Here are a few: Special K, Grape-Nuts, Puffed Wheat, Cheerios,

Cornflakes. You can refer to www.glycemicindex.com for more detailed information.

- Popcorn
- Pasta, gluten free
- Pretzels

You Can Have Vegetables

You really don't need to avoid vegetables. Some are higher glycemic than others such as corn, carrots, beets, and pumpkin. These all have lower glycemic load because they are low in carbohydrates. Bottom line, only avoid potatoes and other starch vegetables that are roots such as yucca.

Fruits to Limit

Fruit is really misunderstood in many nutrition circles. Fruit is sugar, and yes, it has many vitamins; but it is still sugar. Therefore, fruit should not be eaten in unlimited quantities and should be consumed in the earlier part of the day and not at night. Fruit should always be eaten with a dairy product (cottage cheese, white cheese) or with a natural protein (nuts, almonds, etc.) to control the chemical reaction it produces in the body. The following dried fruits must be limited to once a week:

- Dates, dried
- Figs, dried
- Apples, dried
- Apricots, dried
- Golden raisins
- Raisins

Fats to Limit

We talked a lot about the role of fats when it comes to managing our health and the stress response. All fatty foods contain both saturated and unsaturated fatty acids but are usually described as either saturated or unsaturated, depending on the proportions of fatty acids. As we discussed, some fatty acids are called essential fatty acids because our body cannot produce them, and we have to consume them in our diet. These fatty acids are omega-3 and omega-6. In the section on inflammation, we discussed the importance of creating a proper balance of the two fats. Here are the fats to AVOID and limit to create that balance.

- Vegetable oil
- Sunflower oil
- Corn oil
- Soybean oil
- Safflower oil
- Saturated fat
- Margarine
- Sour cream
- Whipping cream
- Hydrogenated or partially hydrogenated vegetable oils (trans fats)

Sugars

When it comes to controlling the stress response, it is important to avoid sugars as much as possible. Insulin management is essential, so it is important to do your best to avoid products that contain sucrose, refined sugar, brown sugar, glucose, glucose syrup, or corn syrup. These concentrated syrups are used widely by the food industry, so it is important to check the food labels. Ingredients on food labels are listed in order, from the most quantity to the least quantity present in the final serving size. If these sugars are near the top of the ingredients list, avoid them altogether. Other sugars to be careful with are:

- Honey. This contains glucose, fructose, and sucrose. Remember, these and all sugars can throw off the chemistry of the diet as we discussed earlier.
- Maltose. This is the kind of sugar that is found in beer. (Sorry, you have to save this for link five).

Protein Food List

As we have discussed, protein is one of the most misunderstood food groups. Protein is absolutely necessary to manage the stress response. Stress breaks the body, and we cannot shut off stress; we can only manage it. This management is about recuperation and repairing the body, and protein is the key.

How Much Protein do you need?

There are new tests being conducted to measure how much protein we need. The indicator amino acid oxidation (IAAO) technique is a more precise new way of measuring individual amino acid and protein requirements of sedentary and active people. The IAAO predicts whole-body protein requirements by measuring the metabolism of a labeled amino acid. Canadian scientists studied human protein requirement using IAAO and determined that the RDA for protein of 0.8 grams per kilogram body weight per day is too low and should be at least 1.2 to 1.4 grams per kilogram body weight per day for sedentary people. Active people should consume 1.4 to 2 grams of protein per kilogram body weight per day. The amount of stress we suffer each day does play a role in the amounts of protein we need.

Measuring

Your hand is a great measurement tool to gauge your protein portion. Usually, you are told to use the palm of your hand; this is too little. I recommend that women measure their protein portion to be the size of one of their hands up to the pinky. Men should consume a portion the same size as one entire hand. It's very unlikely that you will overeat protein, as the body will get full; it's carbohydrates that cause us to overeat.

Good Protein Foods

Fish and Shellfish: Four to five ounces for women and five to seven ounces for men

- All fish and shellfish
- White fish
- Sardines
- Tuna
- Trout
- Herring
- Mackerel
- Salmon

Meat and Poultry: Three to four ounces for women and five to seven ounces for men

- Lean beef
- Turkey breast or leg
- Chicken breast or leg
- Venison
- Rabbit
- Lean pork
- Lean veal
- Lean lamb
- Lean ham

Eggs: Two to three for women and three to four for men.

It has been established that the cholesterol in eggs has no bearing on your blood cholesterol. In fact, my experience is that people's levels of HDL cholesterol improves during the time they consume eggs. Many people don't like too many eggs, so you can create an omelet, adding cheese and ham and using fewer eggs.

Good Dairy Products

- Cottage cheese: Three to four ounces. I find this a great protein source.
- Whey protein powder: Twenty to thirty grams. Whey protein is the collection of globular proteins that can be isolated from whey, a by-product of cheese manufactured from cow's milk. Whey has the highest biological value of any known protein. I have used whey protein for years to help diabetics balance blood sugar and to balance the stress response.
- Cheese: Three to four ounces. Cheese is a great protein as a compliment to salads and vegetables. One to one and a half ounces will give you around six to eight grams of protein.
- Nonfat milk, eight fluid ounces. I have found out that, as we advance into and beyond the second cycle of health, our bodies begin to have more trouble processing milk because of the lactose. If you use milk, it is not a bad idea to get a nonfat/lactose-free milk.
- Yogurt. There is much data on the health benefits of yogurt. Make sure it is without added sugar and fat free. It is always better to use natural yogurt and fresh fruit and a sweetener such as Stevia or Truvia.

Grain Food List

The grains are the main carbohydrates in your meals. You must remember that fruits and vegetables are also carbohydrates. Carbohydrates are not an essential part of the human diet in the same way proteins and some essential fats are because the body can produce all the carbohydrates it needs from proteins and fats. With that being said, we have also discussed the importance of carbohydrates in the diet because it's the brain's only fuel, and that we must protect our muscle, which the body will break down for sugar if it needs to. This is what happens when we don't manage the stress response: The amount of carbohydrates varies in the individual. Myself, I eat many vegetables, but I only need one grain per day at breakfast (phase one), and I never eat fruit. I have incredible health and energy levels. In fact, when I break my regimen and eat more carbohydrates, I get fatigued very quickly.

Measuring

To measure your portion of grains, use your hand; but this time, as a fist. For men, that will be one cup, and women, a little more than a half a cup. It is not an exact science, but it works in the real world. Also, please remember you will not overeat when the stress response is balanced (less hunger/no cravings).

Good Grain Foods

- Sweet potato and yams. These have a higher GL, but can be used in moderation.
- Bread multigrain. One to two slices including rye, barley, and pumpernickel. Bread always has a higher glycemic load, but I have to be realistic that this is one carbohydrate that you can get anywhere with. A trick is to add some fat, preferably some olive oil or peanut butter to lower the GL.
- Cereals. Make sure you find a cereal that is minimally processed and unsweetened (no added sugar). You can lower the GL by adding yogurt instead of milk and add some nuts or ground flaxseed.
- All bran
- Unsweetened muesli
- Oats. Eat steel-cut oats or the old-fashioned rolled oats with the large flakes, not the instant oatmeal, especially the flavored ones—they are

loaded with sugar. Oatmeal is one grain that can give you a variety of different foods such as muffins, bread, pancakes, and biscuits.

- Brown rice. It contains more of the outer husk and is richer in fiber than white rice. The worst rice is sticky rice that is served with sushi. The stickier, the higher the GI.
- Wild rice. This is a great alternative to rice. It is actually not rice, but a grass plant that is very high in fiber and has a great taste.
- Pasta. Look for the pasta made from durum wheat since it contains more fiber than regular white pasta. Buy whole-wheat spaghetti, protein-enriched pasta, and make sure you do not overcook it; best served al dente.
- Barley. Great alternative to rice.
- Buckwheat. My favorite pancakes with sugar-free syrup.
- Bulgur and Couscous
- Quinoa. This is the best grain I have ever come across. It was introduced to me while I was setting up a BioFit Center in Panama. It is high in protein and has a low GL. In the USA, you most likely will have to get it at a health food store. This, to me, is the best alternative to rice.
- Legumes and beans. I put beans in the grain section because they are not a complete protein and are one of the best carbohydrates because they are so high in fiber that they all have a low GI. I find beans work great to balance the stress response in clients who have trouble processing carbohydrates because they help stabilize the blood sugar, thus balancing the stress response.
- Beans of all types. Baked, green, kidneys, lima, pinto, soy—all are good.
- Lentils

Vegetable Food List

Because of the soluble fiber in vegetables, the carbohydrates are absorbed very slowly, converting into sugar without any insulin spike. The non-soluble fiber in the vegetables increases the volume of food and makes you feel full and satisfied without overeating.

Measuring

Once you have set your plate using your hand to measure your protein and fist for the grain, the rest can be filled with vegetables. I just don't believe you have to portion control vegetables and salads. On the stress-response diet, you should not feel hungry between meals (including snacks).

Good Vegetable Foods

Raw and cooked vegetables

- alfalfa sprouts
- bamboo shoots
- broccoli
- cabbage
- carrots
- cauliflower
- celery
- cucumber
- lettuce
- mushrooms
- onions
- peas
- peppers
- radishes
- spinach
- tomatoes
- water chestnuts
- artichokes
- chickpeas
- green beans
- beets
- hummus
- spinach
- zucchini
- pumpkin
- radishes

Fruit Food List

The sugar contained in fruit is fructose. Fructose reacts differently in the body than other kinds of sugar. It is absorbed more slowly and cannot be converted into energy immediately. The GL of fructose is around 19, making it a medium GL carbohydrate. With that being said, fruit is still a sugar. In managing the stress response, it is not recommended to eat unlimited amounts of fruit. I don't recommend eating fruit at night in any of the phases, and no more than two portions per day. I strongly recommend that you eat fruit with either a handful of nuts or with a diary product such as plain yogurt, cottage cheese, or white cheese. Protein helps lower the glycemic load of the fruit, helping to protect the stress response.

Measuring

Keep the portion to one cup or a medium fruit at most. I usually recommend not to use juice unless you're in phase three; but if you do use juice, use a small four-ounce glass and make it fresh. A word of caution: drinking large amounts of juice in the morning can throw off the stress response. *Important rule: Never eat fruit alone, always combine with a healthy fat or protein.*

Good Fruit Foods

- apples
- apricots
- blackberries
- blueberries
- cherries
- grapefruit
- grapes
- kiwi
- lemons
- limes
- melons
- nectarines
- oranges
- peaches
- pears
- pineapple
- plums
- strawberries
- tangerines
- watermelon

Fat Food List

We have talked throughout the book on how important fats are in balancing our inflammation system and maintaining the overall health of the body. All fatty foods contain both saturated and unsaturated fatty acids. What determines if the fat is either saturated or unsaturated are the proportions of the fatty acid present. Unsaturated fats can be further divided into monounsaturated and polyunsaturated fatty acids. As we discussed earlier, the human body can produce some of these fatty acids, but others called essential fatty acids (omega-6 and omega-3) have to be obtained in our diet. The major cause of silent inflammation and diseases associated with it is the imbalance of the essential fatty acids.

Measuring

Fat is our densest source of energy, containing nine calories per gram whereas protein and carbohydrates contain four calories per gram. This makes it important to keep an eye on portion control when it comes to fats. Healthy fats need to be implemented in all the meals as an important factor in managing the stress response.

Good Fat Foods

- almonds, 12-24 nuts
- avocado, ½ of an avocado
- Brazil nuts, 4-5 nuts
- canola oil cold-pressed, 1-2 tsp
- flaxseed oil, 1-2 tsp
- olive oil (extra virgin), 1-2 tsp
- macadamia nuts, 5-6 nuts
- olives, 8-10
- natural peanut butter, 2 tsp
- peanuts, 24
- pistachios, 24
- sunflower seeds, 2 tbsp
- walnuts, 8-12 halves
- butter, 1 pat
- mayonnaise, 2 tsp
- sesame oil, 2 tsp

Snack List

To lower our fat set point and give our metabolism a boost, we must consume healthy snacks between our three main meals. To manage the stress response especially as we enter the second cycle of health, the snacks are essential to maintain our biomarkers. Every client we have over the age of thirty-five years that fail to take an afternoon snack will lose muscle. Our world is just too stressful, and we have to make sure that through our diet, we can recuperate and be healthy. Snacks are a key component to maintaining balance. Here are some ideas:

- Whey Protein Drink. As we discussed in the protein section, this is the best of the best when it comes to an afternoon snack. Whey protein not only maintains muscle and balances stress; it also boosts your productivity by the easy conversion of the whey's amino acids to sugar, giving the brain everything it needs. This is by far the best snack for diabetics and those suffering from metabolic syndrome, as whey will balance out sugar levels. I recommend 20-30 grams per serving. If you're using whey protein in the morning on a phase two, or in the afternoon on a phase three, feel free to add fruit to the mix.
- 3-6 ounces of cottage cheese with 10 almonds
- 1 cup of natural or no-sugar-added yogurt (fruit allowed, depending on phase)
- 12-24 almonds, cashews, whole peanuts—all nuts are good
- 1 tbsp of natural peanut butter with an apple or celery (check phase)
- 1 tbsp natural peanut butter with 3-4 whole-grain crackers (check phase)
- 3-4 ounces of tuna, salmon, or shrimp
- 3-4 ounces of cheese with 10-12 almonds
- One serving of fruit with cheese, yogurt, or nuts (check phase)
- 8-12 olives
- Protein bars (low carbohydrate)
- 1 cup no-sugar-added or sugar-free ice cream or frozen yogurt.
- Others

Note: Snacks are necessary to balance the stress response. Be creative; just follow the guidelines of your particular phase.

Drinks

In "Bio-Link Two: Hydration," you have been taught that when it comes to managing the stress response, hydration and water are as important as exercise and diet. As we will discuss in the next link, the recommendations of eight eight-ounce glasses of water a day is actually low if you have high stress. With that being said, the recommendation on what you should drink will always start with water.

- Water
- Sugar-free drinks such as crystal light, iced tea.
- Diet soda. I recommend only one per day as it contains a lot of sodium and chemicals. Never let soda replace water.
- Coffee (in moderation). Too much coffee can throw off the stress response by increasing adrenaline. But coffee can have many health benefits, everything from fat burning to increasing alertness. I usually have 2-4 cups per day.
- Tea. Tea has been shown to have a number of health benefits, especially green tea. Tea is one of the healthiest drinks to detoxify your body.
- Red wine. There are several studies showing the benefits of a glass or two of red wine daily. I usually don't recommend alcohol for those on phase one menus, but a glass once in a while will not hurt. This is the drink I opt for in social situations.

Note: All other alcohol should be avoided unless it is your junk night. I also caution you on drinking milk as it contains sugar as lactose, and most adults have trouble (whether they know it or not) digesting it. Also, avoid fruit juices after breakfast and all canned fruit juice (again, it's better to eat the fruit). Avoid beer unless you find a low-carb beer and as with wine once in a while.

Fiber: Two Sides of the Story

Dietary fiber plays a very important role in managing the stress response. Fiber is found only in plant foods. It's a structural and storage form of carbohydrate and is not digested as it passes through the human digestive system. Fiber is classified by its ability to dissolve in water, and there are two types: water soluble and water insoluble.

- Soluble fibers come primarily from beans, fruits, and whole grains. Soluble fiber can be dissolved in water and include plant materials such as gums, mucilages, pectin, and some hemicelluloses.
- Insoluble fibers come mainly from vegetables, beans, whole wheat, and fruit skins. Insoluble fiber doesn't dissolve in water and includes lignins, cellulose, and some hemicelluloses.

Fiber Benefits

Even though there are two types of fiber, they both work to improve the job of the intestines, although in different ways. The water-soluble fibers are generally sticky and viscous and slow the down the movement of food through the digestive tract. Water insoluble fibers act like stool softeners and bulk formers and keep things moving through our system. Fiber benefits include:

- Controlling and preventing diabetes. The presence of water-soluble fiber in the diet helps reduce the absorption of sugars and starches from the small intestine into the bloodstream. This helps maintain control of blood sugar levels by keeping it from raising and dropping drastically. This also helps with stress response by controlling the hormone insulin.
- Intestinal health. Fiber promotes regularity and has been shown to promote digestive system health. By decreasing the time it takes to move the food through the intestines, water insoluble fibers improve elimination, and at the same time, flush carcinogens, bile acids, and cholesterol out of the system. These actions help alleviate constipation and diverticular disease.
- Decreasing cardiovascular diseases. The body manufactures the majority of its cholesterol in the intestines and bile acids recycle the cholesterol. Water-soluble fibers have a cholesterol-lowering effect by binding to bile acids and keeping the cholesterol from recycling.
- Weight control. Dietary fiber plays an important role when it comes to overall weight management. Fiber helps to slow the time it takes for your stomach to empty; you feel full longer and eat less.

How Much Fiber

Generally, the stress-response diet is built around fiber, and we need fiber to stay healthy and prevent disease. Adults need to eat at least twenty-five grams of fiber per day. Many experts agree that we should increase that number to thirty to thirty-five grams per day. High fruit fiber diets were linked to lower blood pressure and abdominal fat. High vegetable fiber diets were related to lower blood pressure and levels of homocysteine—a chemical linked to blood vessel inflammation. Each increment of five grams of fiber intake provided additional health benefits. In the United States, the average adult only consumes fifteen grams of fiber per day.

The Other Side of the Fiber Story

Can we eat too much fiber? The answer is yes, especially if you are a male over age forty. When vegetarians with high-fiber diets (fifty grams) were compared to Western low-fat diets (twenty grams fiber), vegetarians had lower testosterone levels. Testosterone is the main male hormone that keeps the biomarkers (muscle) healthy. When the data was closely analyzed, the higher the fiber intake, the lower the testosterone production. The reason for the lower testosterone levels was that this high fiber was binding testosterone and not allowing enough free testosterone for the body to be anabolic. So fiber is needed for optimal health, but there is also too much of a good thing and it can have adverse effects on your health.

Metabolic Eating

One of the tricks I have learned over the years is what I call metabolic eating, meaning, the order in which we consume our meals and the type of snacks to control hunger and increase fat burning. We covered this in the protein section when I mentioned that the liver converts amino acids from proteins into blood sugar, which manages the stress response and prevents hunger. A simple but very effective strategy is to take a whey protein supplement (fifteen to thirty grams) between meals, which will prevent hunger and overeating.

Another trick is the order in which you eat your meals. This metabolic eating order will make it so you consume fewer calories and rev up the metabolism.

- Start with a soup. Follow your phase guidelines and order a soup or make a healthy soup. When in a restaurant, if your soup has ingredients in it that you are not allowed, simply eat around them and consume the broth.

- Eat a hearty salad. When following the stress-response menu many times, we are increasing the protein in the diet. Studies show that when you eat more protein to keep the alkaline in the body balanced, we need to consume more vegetables. The stress-response diet is built to do this. When in restaurants or at home keep the use of dressings to a minimum. I recommend you use olive oil,vinegar, salt and pepper to dress your salads. Balsamic vinergar is particularly healthy for you.
- Consume your protein with your vegetables. It is all right to eat lentils and other beans along with the protein.
- Eat the starch last. What causes most weight gain is the amount of carbohydrates we consume, and it is also what imbalances the stress response. Eating the pasta, whole-grain bread, healthy rice, sweet potato, etc., at the end ensures that you won't overeat and lowers the glycemic index.
- Fruit or sugar-free dessert. This goes without saying. It is great to have a piece of dark chocolate at the end of a great meal.

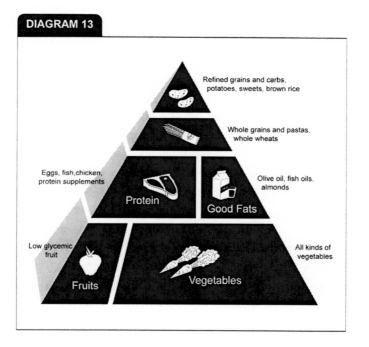

DIAGRAM 13

Refined grains and carbs, potatoes, sweets, brown rice

Whole grains and pastas, whole wheats

Eggs, fish,chicken, protein supplements

Protein

Olive oil, fish oils, almonds

Good Fats

Low glycemic fruit

All kinds of vegetables

Fruits

Vegetables

Top: to be consumed only on "Junk Night": sugar, white bread, white potatoes, white rice, white flour, trans fats, straches.

Next tier: grains, wheat, pasta, wild rice or brown rice, long-grain rice, basmati, quinoa, whole grain products, breads, and low glycemic fruit.

Next tier: unsaturated fat, olive oil, nuts and seeds, canola oil, oily fish,
    coconut oil and in limited amounts, saturated fats, butter, and fatty cheese.
Next tier: protein—chicken, fish, meat, game, eggs, yogurt, cheese, cottage
    cheese, and whey protein drinks.
Last tier: Fruit, legumes and all types of vegetables and beans.

Eduardo's Story

Eduardo is a fifty-three-year-old high-level business executive with
above normal stress. He had been recently diagnosed with early stages of
type 2 diabetes. He was brought to one of the BioFit Centers from his
company to help him get healthy so he could pass the company's yearly
physical examination. Eduardo's company's medical director came with him
and explained that he had to get his weight down or he could lose his job.
Needless to say, Eduardo was truly motivated.

In Eduardo's first follow-up, the results were amazing. He had gained
ten lbs of muscle, decreased seven lbs of fat, and dropped 4 percent of body
fat. I was happy, but the problem was he had gained 3.3 pounds of weight.
I personally didn't have a problem with this, but the medical director of the
company went crazy. They were so upset that they threatened to pull their
corporate account from us.

The team (along with me) panicked. We took drastic measures and
changed Eduardo's program. We cut the diet by 500 calories, stopped the
weight training, and started increasing his exercise with boxing and other
calorie-burning exercises so he wouldn't gain muscle. In thirty days, we had
another follow-up, and we wanted to be ready.

When Eduardo weighed in, we were all excited because he had lost three
pounds. Then we received the real news. He had lost weight, but his muscle
dropped eight pounds and his fat increased over six pounds, and even though
he weighed less on the scale, his body fat increased 3 percent.

I was so upset with myself because I knew better than to cut his calories
and increase his training. I threw off his stress response, and the rest was
history. The scale is the worst measurement of any true wellness program.
I immediately put him back on the program that had worked in the
beginning by increasing his calories and modifying the workout back into
his zones. I swore to myself from that day forward I would never make that
mistake again. It's important that the medical field begin to embrace a new
measurement guideline for health because the scale and the BMI just don't
give us the truth.

Conclusion

The causes of obesity in these modern times are psychological and physiological. The physiological part we have discussed in detail. We must understand that stress plays a crucial role in the way our body performs. Our stress response isn't designed to work in this technological age of 24/7 stress. We cannot shut the stress off, but we can manage how our bodies will handle it from a day-to-day basis, and our diet is one of the keys.

When it comes to the psychological cause of obesity, we went into much detail about that in part 3 of this book on "The Mind." When you order a burger and fries, for a mere twenty-five cents, you can supersize it. It will double your fries and drink! Why not? It is quite a deal. America is the land of the giants when it comes to portion size and the amount of food we can pile on our plates. This became so evident to me as the last six to seven years I have been living and traveling outside the United States. When I come home, there is no way I can possibly finish a restaurant-size order. Meanwhile, all around, people are not only finishing everything on their plate (remember, "Part Three: The Mind"), they are also ordering dessert. Penn State researchers found that portion sizes in the United States are, on the average, 100 percent larger and contain 26 percent more calories than in other countries. I can tell you from personal experience that this is an absolute fact.

It is crucial to understand that our diet plays a major role in how we handle the stress response. Wrong diet combined with too much food will throw off the stress response, causing you to be hungrier, thus causing you to eat more. A viscous cycle for sure, but a cycle that can be broken with this very program. It is important to understand "Bio Link One: Meals," as the more you understand, the easier it is to take control. Link One, Meals is the first link of the chain of health. Lets now take a look at link Two, Hydration.

Chapter Seventeen

Bio-Link Two: Hydration why drinking is so important

Water, air, and cleanliness are the chief articles in my pharmacopoeia.
—Napoleon I

The stress-response diet program considers hydration to be so important that it represents one of the five bio-links to health. When it comes to balancing the stress response, drinking enough water is essential, not just a good idea. The fact is you can be eating a perfect diet and following the perfect exercise regimen, but without proper hydration, you will not manage stress. Our bodies need to stay hydrated, especially if we have high stress levels and as we get older. As we age, our bodies' thirst mechanism begins to slow down despite the fact that our fluid output stays the same. If we don't replenish the lost liquid, we become dehydrated, and our body functions, including our metabolism, will slow down.

You can live for a long time without food, but not without water. Water makes up more than 70 percent of our body's tissue. Water helps regulate body temperature (biomarker no. 10), and it carries nutrients and oxygen to cells, including our brain. Water is what removes waste byproducts from our bodies and cushions our joints while protecting our organs and tissues. "Link Two: Hydration" is a key link when it comes to the stress response.

The Stress Response and Hydration

When it comes to managing the stress response, drinking enough water is as important as exercise or the diet. As we have discussed throughout the book, our stress response is part of our survival mechanism. It is literally built-in. So let's take a scenario where you're at your desk and you get upset with someone. Your body releases the stress hormones to prepare you take action. What action can you take? You cannot jump over the desk and attack the person, and you cannot go running down the street like a crazy person. You cannot take action, so what happens to the stress hormones? Well, they turn into toxins and cause a breakdown of the body while increasing free radicals. This will, over time, cause you to become ill, tired, and completely run-down. What is the solution? You must stimulate your lymph system and simply drinking enough water does this. Becoming hydrated is essential to maintain good health.

Are You Dehydrated?

The answer is simple. If you are not drinking at least ten to twelve eight-ounce glasses of water daily, you are most likely dehydrated. Forget that old eight glasses of water daily, there is just too much stress nowadays. It is so important to drink enough because even slight dehydration can throw your body off. A lack of adequate water intake can lead to headaches, sluggishness, fatigue, dry skin, and unmanaged stress. More severe dehydration can affect blood pressure, circulation, digestion, kidney function, and nearly all basic body processes. It can also cause loss of balance, extreme weakness, and even death. Many of the aliments that elderly patients (especially seventy years and older) are treated for can literally be caused by dehydration and avoided with proper hydration.

Water and Fat Loss

As crazy as it sounds, drinking water helps you eliminate excess water. In the same way that your body holds on to fat when you eat too little, the body holds on to water when you do not drink enough of it. If the body holds on to water, the result will be a bloated feeling and appearance plus a few pounds on the scale of water weight. The best diuretic is drinking plenty of water each day. This not only helps our body function at optimal levels, but it also helps us lose excess weight and eat less. Most people get hunger signals prematurely because they are dehydrated. They believe they are hungry so they eat, when in reality, they were dehydrated. Bottom line, drink water and lose weight. Drinking water also replaces calorie-containing beverages and may aid in energy expenditure. Drinking as little as a half a liter of water actually increases the neurotransmitters that signal fat release from the fat cells. When researchers measured people's metabolic rate before and after drinking about sixteen ounces of water, they found a rise in calorie-burning capability. So please drink water if you want to lose weight.

Hydrating the Body

The initial phase of hydration is characterized by one simple act, running to the bathroom very frequently. This can be uncomfortable and inconvenient at first, but it lasts only a few days or a week. Once you get over this initial period, the trips to the restroom are regulated and become less frequent.

Let me explain why this occurs. The one thing that we all have in common is we are all highly affected by stress. When we experience the stress response, our bodies react by releasing the hormones to set our bodies into action. As we have discussed, these hormones are designed for our survival and to make us fight or flight. Taking action is not an option as we live in societies that demand certain standards of behavior. When our bodies are not able to release the effect of the fight-or-flight hormones through some type of action, they become toxins in our body, creating illness, fatigue, and tight muscles.

When you begin hydrating the body, you stimulate the lymphatic system and your kidneys, allowing the body to begin the process of ridding itself of toxins and poisons. The toxins are eliminated through the kidneys, bladder and urine. This is the reason why, when we begin to hydrate, we run to the bathroom very often. This will settle down in a week or so, but you will start to notice the more stress you experience, the more you will be going to the bathroom. This is a good thing.

When I do corporate seminars for executives, all of them are living under great amounts of stress. Before I teach them about nutrition or exercise, I will focus on hydration; it is one of the easiest stress management tools around. I have found that most people experience fatigue around 3:00

p.m. This happens in part because of the accumulation of stress that occurs during the day. In other words, an accumulation of stress that has occurred during the day leads to an accumulation of toxins in the body. Most people will grab a coffee or a soft drink when they hit this wall and are tired and stressed. Caffeine can actually cause the body even more stress, and that means more toxins.

The secret is to stop your activities the moment you feel fatigued and drink three to four glasses of water to stimulate your lymphatic system. This will help rid your body of toxins and poisons. You will immediately feel better, and you will notice an increase in physical and mental energy. This is a valuable tool for those working hard to maintain a peak performance throughout the day. Give it a try and see for yourself, I guarantee you will be amazed.

Hydrating Guidelines

I have worked with many clients over the last twenty-eight years and have found that the following guidelines apply for most people:

- When fully hydrated, the average female will drink around three quarts of water per day.
- When fully hydrated, the average male will drink around one gallon of water per day.

These are just guidelines; not all individuals are the same. It is important to understand that we must drink enough water to manage the stress response. One way to easily know if you are hydrated is by the color of your urine. You should drink enough water to keep your urine colorless. Dark yellow urine is a sure sign of ensuing dehydration. If you have trouble drinking water, you can try these ideas:

- Sugar-free drink mixes such as crystal light for example
- Adding lemon or lime to flavor the water
- Tea, no sugar added

Important

The hydration process can take a couple weeks. After this period, the body will become hydrated and then literally begin asking you for water. In other words, you will get thirsty. DO NOT force the process of hydration. The following schedule works great in getting the body hydrated:

Week one: Drink one quart of water each day. Use a quart-size container to help you measure.

Week two: Drink two quarts of water. Drink one quart in the morning and one quart in the afternoon.

Week three: Drink three quarts of water. Drink one and a half quarts in the morning and one and half quarts in the afternoon.

Week four: Your body will be hydrated and it will literally dictate the right amount of water for you. Always use a container that you can measure the amount to keep you on track (water bottle). Monitor the color of your urine. Staying hydrated will just become natural.

If you are never thirsty (especially if you are in your seventies or older), this is a great trick. Drink two glasses of water before each meal and every snack. This will give you ten glasses of water a day. Then make sure you drink three glasses, one before exercising, one during, and one after. This will guarantee that you are hydrated. When you are fully hydrated, you will not only manage the stress response, but you will also eat less in your meals and speed up your metabolism.

Chapter Eighteen

Bio-Link Three: Circulation
Knowing your Fat Burning Zone

"Exercise is the chief source of improvement in our faculties"
—Hugh Blair

Miguel's Story

Miguel was a fifty-two-year-old businessman who came to me as a referral from his cardiologist. Three months earlier, Miguel had gone to the hospital because of chest pain. While in the hospital, it was discovered that Miguel had several blockages in his arteries and had to have a procedure to open them up. Miguel received three stents and was now looking for answers on why this had happened. The reason Miguel was looking for an answer was because he thought he was following the perfect lifestyle program so he wondered how could this have happened?

Miguel had been a competitive athlete in track and field while he was in college and had been exercising for over thirty years. He had a very balanced diet, eating several meals a day consisting of lean proteins, vegetables, fruits, and healthy whole-grain starches. Miguel did have some visible excess fat around his midsection, but he was not overweight at all. Miguel's training regimen was very extensive. Before he was hospitalized, he was running one to two hours every morning for six days per week. He was competing in full marathons and would regularly push his body to the limits as he had done in his younger days when he was an athlete.

I received several of Miguel's tests from his doctor, and I noticed that in one of the previous exams, he had an elevated C-reactive protein indicating increased inflammation in his body. I ran a cardio-metabolic stress test to get Miguel's proper aerobic zone and his VO_2 max. I also did an advanced composition test to get his muscle-to-fat ratios and an accurate body composition. When I gave Miguel his results and my recommendations, he was not at all too happy. Even though he was not overweight, his body composition was poor with excess fat and a low 3.6:1 muscle-to-fat ratio indicating a large breakdown in the biomarkers. His cardio-metabolic test wasn't any better, showing a low VO_2 max and a low aerobic zone.

The exercise program I put Miguel on consisted of two days a week of resistance training to improve his biomarkers and walking in his zone to improve his aerobic capacity. Even though Miguel was not happy, he trusted my recommendations and complied perfectly. In sixty days, his life had changed dramatically. His muscle-to-fat ratio was now 5:1, and he had enormous energy and had lost all excess fat. His VO_2 max improved, allowing him to start interval training in his zone. Miguel was now in the best shape he had been in the last twenty years and still finds it hard to believe he accomplished all of this without killing himself.

Miguel's story is a common theme at the BioFit Centers around the world. "Link Three: Circulation" is about doing aerobic exercise. Aerobic exercise is necessary to manage the stress response and is the best option for people after the second cycle of health to improve their cardiac condition.

Consistent aerobic exercise is a major key in correcting hormone balance, especially leptin and insulin hormones, which play a key role in fat burning. The biggest challenge is that most of us are like Miguel, and we have no idea what aerobic exercise really means. When we hear this term, we immediately think of jogging, running, spinning, or jumping up and down in an aerobics class. Running, spinning, and endurance sports are not aerobic exercise. They are cardiovascular exercises. In other words, they require our heart and lungs to perform under extremely high intensity. This "no pain, no gain" approach to exercise throws the stress response into complete chaos after age thirty-five. Let's look at the difference between aerobic and cardiovascular exercise.

Aerobic versus Cardiovascular

Aerobic exercise is not running, spinning, or playing sports. It is when you exercise within your specific aerobic heart rate zone that you allow your body to use fat as fuel. One of the questions I ask in my wellness seminars is this: "Is there a difference between aerobic and cardiovascular exercise?" On an average, about 90 percent of the people will answer no. Most of us think aerobic and cardiovascular exercise is the same thing. Most people (especially baby boomers) believe that if they are working up a sweat and have a soaring heart rate, they are doing aerobic exercise. Simply not true!

True aerobic exercise is done in a heart rate zone that is tested with a cardio-metabolic stress test that determines the VO_2 max. When you exercise in that aerobic zone heart rate for a period of time, the body will build up oxygen. Aerobic simply means "in the presence of oxygen." In the stress-response program, "Bio-Link Three: Circulation" refers to this type of aerobic exercise. Building up oxygen is the primary key for the body to burn fat and the body's ability to burn fat is the key to longevity, optimal health, great energy levels, and permanent weight loss.

Cardiovascular exercise, on the other hand, is any type of activity that makes your heart and lungs work at high-intensity levels for an undetermined period of time. Cardiovascular exercise is not necessarily aerobic, since the presence of oxygen is not always possible during high-intensity activity.

As we enter the second cycle of health (thirty-five to forty-five years), our preconceived ideas of exercise need to change. The "no pain, no gain" mentality needs to be replaced by "no brain, no gain" when it comes to exercise and managing the stress response. As in Miguel's case, when you exercise too hard, it can be worse for you than not exercising at all. In order to see results from exercise after the second cycle of health, we have to strive for consistency rather than intensity.

The Stress Response and Exercise

As I mentioned earlier, we have all been taught that the more calories we burn during the exercise, the better. That is true when we are younger and in the first cycle of health below thirty-five years of age. After we enter the second cycle, the body doesn't react the same way toward stress anymore. This is why many professional athletes retire after age thirty-five. They haven't lost their skills, they have lost their ability to recuperate. When we exercise, our bodies cannot tell the difference between a spinning class and running from a pack of wolves. The stress response kicks in for the body to take action releasing the necessary hormones for the body to perform the required physical activity. Once this finalizes, these stress hormones drop.

The key to exercise recuperation is the rebalance of the stress response. When I work with professional athletes, this is key for optimal performance. The success of exercise is not how hard you push, it is about the body's ability to recuperate from that exercise session. When we are young, our bodies recuperate quite easily because of the body's ability to handle stress. Aerobic exercise is a vital key for overall health, aging of the body, and managing the stress response.

The Aerobic Zone

It is important not to feel exhausted from your exercise program. It is vital if you are in the second cycle of health or older to stay within your zone during exercise. Exercise is a must if you want to create optimal health and longevity. When older people exercise three or more times a week, they are less likely to develop Alzheimer's and other types of dementia, according to a study that adds to the growing body of evidence that staying active can help keep the body healthy and the mind sharp.

Researchers found that healthy people who reported exercising regularly had a 30 to 40 percent lower risk of dementia. The study published in the Annals of Internal Medicine reached no conclusions about whether certain types of exercise helped more than others, but researchers said even light activity, such as walking seemed to help. This is aerobic exercise, not running and getting yourself out of breath. Dr. Wayne McCormick, a University of Washington geriatrician who was one of the study's authors said, "The surprising finding for us was that it actually didn't take much exercise to have this effect." I can tell you for a fact that this is true. For many years in the United States, my client's average age was seventy years old; I was one of the first to work with seventy-, eighty-, and ninety-year-old clients. When I start them on a program of weight-bearing exercise and aerobic training, they would improve all functions in as little as two weeks.

Mild exercise such as walking in your aerobic zone has a profound effect on managing the stress response. When you manage the stress response, the cells can easily utilize fat for energy, and that reverses the biological age. Remember, your biological age is determined by how your body is producing energy; is it burning fat properly? The key to fat burning is oxygen, and the key to building up oxygen is aerobic exercise. Exercising too hard actually ages the body and causes you to store fat. Yes, if you exercise too hard, you will get fatter. Just look at many middle-age runners; they are exercising, but never reduce their waist size. Bottom line, they are not burning fat.

When you exercise, it is essential to remain in your aerobic exercise zone for at least thirty to forty minutes to get the most out of the exercise session. This should be done at least three times per week; but honestly, you cannot over train in your zone.

Calculating Your Aerobic Zone

Amanda's Story

Amanda was a forty-five-year-old mother of three that had been in a training program for over four months with a personal trainer. In that time period, Amanda told me she had only lost about six pounds, even though she was following a rather strict menu and training hard four to five times a week with her trainer. Amanda was complaining about more than not getting results. She was complaining of always being sore and lately, had bad cravings for sweets especially on the days she worked out. Amanda was also complaining of being so tired in the afternoon she could barely function at work.

When I reviewed her program, I found out she was in a boot-camp type of workout that was intense; but as she stated, it was monitored so she would be in her correct workout zones. Amanda's trainer used two common formulas to determine her zone, and those are:

$$220\text{-age} \times 0.65 = \text{FBR (maximum fat-burning rate)}$$
$$220\text{-age} \times 0.85 = \text{ATR (anaerobic threshold rate)}$$

With this formula, Amanda's trainer put her zone at FBR = 113 and ATR = 148, and he trained Amanda at the top end of her zone, close to the full hour of the class.

When we tested Amanda with the cardio-metabolic stress test (bio-energy), we received our answers quickly as to why she was feeling so badly. Her actual zones were FBR = 85 and ATR = 112, so her aerobic zone was 85 beats per minute to 112 beats per minute. Amanda also had a very low VO_2 max, so her body was literally unable to burn fat for energy. To make matters worse, Amanda's boot-camp training was making her fatter as her calculated FBR was 113, and in reality, her ATR or her max was below that at 112. While she was being monitored during her workouts, the zones were so far off that her body was in a state of extreme stress, throwing off her stress response and causing her symptoms of fatigue and intense cravings.

We adjusted Amanda's exercise program and incorporated her proper zones and within the first thirty days, she lost six pounds of fat and gained one pound of muscle. Her energy was back up and most important she was actually enjoying her new exercise regimen.

Amanda's story is common to us when we test people at the BioFit Centers. We have been taught to push hard and sweat a lot, and this just doesn't work as we go into the second cycle of health above age thirty-five; the body just cannot handle the stress. I recommend that you get tested at a BioFit Center. You may find our center's location in the United States and other countries by going to www.biofitprogram.com. I recommend that you contact one of our BioFit counselors online if you want to get tested and go on the program.

For those who cannot get tested, I have used this formula with great success for clients around the world.

1. 220 - your age = your max heart rate (MHR)
2. MHR x 60% = low-end fat-burning rate (FBR)
3. MHR x 70% = high-end FBR
4. 60%-70% of MHR = Fat-burning zone
5. MHR x 85% = anaerobic threshold rate (ATR)

I recommend if you are taking blood pressure medications or any type of beta-blocker, drop all the above calculations by 5 percent. For example, MHR multiplied by 55 percent, instead of 60 percent for the low end of the FBR, and so on.

BioFit aerobic training

The exercise we do must help us manage stress, not increase it. When you perform your exercise, you must wear a heart monitor. Your heart rate is one of the best indicators of how your body is handling the stress response. The key to everything healthy, including longevity, is getting our body to burn fat properly. To get our body to burn fat, we must exercise in our fat-burning zone, and we must improve our body's ability to burn fat by improving our VO_2 max and the amount of oxygen in our cells. When your heart rate goes above your ATR for longer than a few minutes, you cause your body to break down, and it increases the level of free-radical damage to the body. When your heart rate is below your FBR, your exercise will be inefficient, and you will be wasting your time. The heart monitor is a key tool to allow you to train properly. Your heart rate will change on a regular basis according to the time of day, stress levels, and environment (especially when you travel). When you use a heart rate monitor, you are creating a perfect exercise condition that not only will manage the stress response, but will also help you obtain all your weight loss goals. Biological age is determined by how well the body produces energy, and to reverse the biological age and increase energy levels, you have to optimize your aerobic exercise. This is done through interval training.

BioFit interval training

At the BioFit Centers, we implement interval training to get the fastest results in the shortest period of time. Interval training is when you alternate training between your FBR (maximum Fat burning rate) and ATR (anaerobic threshold rate) to maximize the cell's ability to burn fat. When you push the heart rate to your maximum rate (ATR), you are on the top of your zone; and when you are at the bottom of your zone (FBR), the body will recuperate from the interval.

Interval training works in the following method:

- Warm-up period is about five minutes in duration. After a couple of minutes, work your way up to your FBR.
- After the five-minute warm-up, push yourself to your ATR and stay there for one to two minutes.
- After the two minutes at your ATR, push yourself really hard for thirty seconds going above your zone. Yes, I have said that going outside your zone is harmful, but a short burst or push is great to strengthen the mitochondria. Extended time outside the zone causes the body to produce energy anaerobically—without oxygen—and this is harmful if done for too long, a short period of thirty to forty seconds will give you great results.
- After your anaerobic burst, slow your way down to where you almost stop the exercise and get back to your FBR so your body can recover. Stay in the FBR rate for three to four minutes. If you need it longer, do it; intervals only work if there is sufficient recovery time.
- After you have recovered, shoot back up to your ATR and repeat the process. I recommend thirty minutes to one hour, three to six times per week.

Fat Burning

At the BioFit Centers, we have thousands of clients that get fast and spectacular results with interval training, and we have other clients who just want to keep it simple. These clients are told to maintain their heart rate between their FBR and ATR and simply walk or bike, etc. It doesn't have to be complicated, but it does have to be monitored. There is nothing wrong with maintaining a steady rate for thirty to sixty minutes, three to six days a week. Actually, you can do aerobic exercise every day and not overdo it, as long as you wear your heart monitor. Your heart rate will set the intensity of your training. You cannot go wrong.

Athletic Training: No Pain, No Gain

After age thirty-five, when you exercise above your ATR, you can cause extended damage to your body and your health. When we are in the first cycle of health (below twenty to thirty-five), our body will recuperate and balance the stress response very efficiently. After age thirty-five, the body doesn't recuperate and the intense exercise will actually cause the body to store fat and age rather quickly. This is why many athletes, both professional and amateur, will have a lot of injuries after age thirty-five. The truth is to win a race you will have to spend an extended time in your ATR, but the fact will remain that this is not good for your long-term health. I suggest that if you are over thirty-five and want to compete in sports, get a sports nutritionist to prescribe the right menu and supplements to make sure the body will recuperate. At BioFit, we train many professional athletes, and the diet is as important as the training especially as they get older. One nutritional mistake and the training will be useless as the body cannot balance the stress response.

Conclusion

- Try to get a metabolic stress test or a bio-energy test to know your real scientific aerobic zones. The BioFit Center is located in Miami Beach, Fl. And Panama City, Panama and are designed to create a complete program tailored specifically for you to obtain optimal health.
- Interval training can speed up your results and make the exercise much more fun.

- Buy yourself a heart-rate monitor and never exercise without it. Don't guess; know that you are getting the perfect workout.
- Studies have shown that to maintain good health, we need to exercise six hours per week. I agree that this is a good minimum to manage the stress response. Out of the six hours, three to four hours need to be monitored aerobic exercise.
- Make sure to retest your bio-energy or cardio-metabolic stress test every six months to a year. Your zones will change as you progress.

Chapter Nineteen

Bio-Link Four: Lean Body mass
Resistance Training
The Secret Fountain of Youth

"Opposition is a natural part of life. Just as we develop our physical muscles through overcoming opposition—such as lifting weights—we develop our character muscles by overcoming challenges and adversity."
—Stephen R. Covey

Alan's Story

Alan is a seventy-nine-year-old client that was brought to me by his daughter who was worried because he was tired all the time and didn't want to leave the house. Alan was a relatively healthy seventy-nine-year-old but, lately, admitted he wasn't himself. Alan had been active all his life but, recently, was experiencing such fatigue that not only did he not exercise, but also didn't really want to do anything but sleep and watch TV.

When I did Alan's workup, not surprisingly, I found a low ratio of muscle to fat; he was 2.5:1 (Ideally, we want 5:1). I contacted Alan's cardiologist to set up a physical and get a medical clearance for him to start his exercise regimen. After a few days, Alan's cardiologist called my assistant and gave orders that Alan could walk, but he didn't believe he could do any other type of training. I personally called Alan's doctor to see what the reason was for not letting Alan participate in an exercise program. The doctor told me that Alan was in good health and passed his stress test without any problem, but he was seventy-nine years old, and how can a man his age do weight training?

This is common among the medical field. They will recommend exercise, but that usually means walking, and not resistance training. I explained to the doctor that when we have a client over the age of sixty-five at BioFit we train them with three different protocols.

1. We use light resistant training called functional training (this can be getting out of a chair), and we work to increase their flexibility. This exercise is designed to restore their muscle and lean body mass.
2. We will work on their balance with different routines. As we age, falling is one of our greatest fears. Many elderly clients are afraid to be active because they fear falling.
3. We will do a series of exercises for cognitive function, making the brain work and react to exercises. These exercises can be as easy as playing catch.

After explaining to Alan's physician BioFit's protocols of training, I received the medical release to start his exercise program. Within two weeks, Alan's daughter approached me and told me she was absolutely shocked by her father's results. This was the best she had seen him in the last ten years. This is very common with my seventy-plus clients; they will show dramatic results in just a few weeks. After just thirty days, Alan's muscle-to-fat ratio was up to 4:1 ratios. He was a completely different man from when he had first walked into the Center. Recently, Alan's cardiologist has reduced his medications for his brand-new biologically younger body.

According to the ten biomarkers and Drs. Evan and Rosenberg's scientific studies, lean body mass (muscle) is the key in achieving optimal health, reducing your biological age, and achieving permanent weight (fat) loss. Muscle mass determines your basal metabolic rate (BMR). The more muscle mass you have, the higher your metabolism and the more calories your body burns at rest.

You know my personal story of struggling during the first half of my life with weight loss. I would lose weight and then gain it all back, plus a few more pounds. My problem, like so many people, was keeping the weight off. During this time, I discovered the wonderful powers of building muscle. My body literally changed from being obese to looking like a bodybuilding champion in very little time. During those early years, I was shocked at how my body reacted to resistance training. That is when I realized that the key to achieving permanent weight loss and achieving optimal health was the creation and preservation of the body's lean body mass.

During the early eighties, when I started bodybuilding, I realized that not many people were lifting weights, not even athletes. In those years, there were so many misconceptions about the effects of resistance training that most people and coaches stayed away from it. Athletes believed that weight training would make them slow and muscle bound (Tiger Woods is one of the first athletes who shattered that myth). Women were also very fearful of weight training because they didn't want to "look like men" or "get bulky." Active adults would fear getting injured; they believed after a certain age, it is not possible to do resistance-training workouts. Many doctors were also very misinformed on resistance training; they would tell their patients with high blood pressure, diabetes, bad backs, and other aliments that weights would be dangerous for them (unfortunately, even with all the science available, I still hear these type of statements from some doctors today).

The absolute truth is without resistance training, there is no possible way to keep your biomarkers healthy. I was one of the first to incorporate resistance training to create permanent weight (fat) loss. Many weight-loss programs frown upon weight training because the scale may not have the drastic change that we are programmed to believe it should have. In other words, you won't lose a lot of weight on the scale, even though you will fit perfectly into your clothes and look incredible in the mirror or a bathing suit. I was also one of the first to incorporate weight training with clients seventy years and older. It is an essential element to be able to lower the individual's biological age and restore them to optimal health. I also know firsthand that if you suffer from back pain, you MUST do weight training. In 1985, I had my spine fused in my lower back. I spent months in a body cast and in the hospital doing rehab. Twenty-four years later, I still have what would be considered a bad back; but I am pain free and suffer zero aliments as long as I weight train. The moment I stop, within a few days, the back will act up. The answer is simple; muscle is the key. Let's take a look at the complete benefits of this link.

Resistance Training and Creating Permanent Weight Loss

Any bodybuilder will tell you that the biggest challenge in the sport is "cutting up" for a contest. This is when a bodybuilder will take his body fat down to the lowest possible percentage to be able to display their physique on stage. The challenge for bodybuilders is how to lose fat and maintain their muscle mass. It is the same challenge when it comes to any type of weight-loss program. When we diet, we invariably lose muscle mass (the stress response is thrown off with signal of less food) when we lose body weight, which affects the ten biomarkers and causes decrease in strength and aerobic capacity. When the aerobic capacity drops, the body will lose its ability to burn fat so any further weight loss will be muscle.

Researchers at the Washington University School of Medicine in St. Louis proved the weight-loss effect of dieting. In a one-year study of middle-aged adults (second cycle of health), researchers found that people who lost weight through calorie restriction decreased 3.5 percent in lean mass (muscle), 6.9 percent in thigh muscle volume, 7.2 percent in knee flexion strength, and 6.8 percent in aerobic capacity. The bottom line here is that the calorie-restricted group lost weight but also increased their aging process and destroyed their metabolism and they have zero chance to keep the weight off.

On the other hand, the people in the study who lost weight through exercise alone lost 10 percent of body weight, but had no decrease in muscle size or strength. They also improved a whopping 30 percent in aerobic capacity, thus lowering their biological age and maximizing their fat-burning capabilities. Again, much of this that I am teaching you I know to be true from personal experience, but now science is backing up what I have taught for thirty years—Diets don't work.

Muscle and the Metabolism

How does your lean body mass (muscle) influence your entire metabolism? The basal metabolic rate (BMR) is the main factor determining how many calories your body will burn every day. Your lean body mass will determine how strong your BMR will be. Remember, we burn 90 percent of our calories in the lean body mass; and the BMR not only will determine your daily caloric expenditure, but it is also critical for fat gains and losses, particularly in the abdomen. The nervous system sends a steady stream of impulses to the tissues that help control metabolism and the rate at which you burn calories. This process works like a furnace; turn up the thermostat (muscle), the more heat will be generated. In your body, the higher the setting on the thermostat, the more calories you burn every day.

Muscle is made up of active cells, and it maintains a slight contraction even at rest. This means that even a slight increase in muscle mass will cause your body to use more energy throughout the day, thus raising your BMR. On the other hand, body fat is made up of inactive cells, serving as a storage depot for more fat. So now you can understand what happened on your last attempt to lose weight on a calorie-restricted diet. You lost weight, but without exercise, it will be muscle weight. This then lowers the number of calories your body burns, lowering your BMR and your metabolism. Invariably, your body believes it is in starvation, so it has to replace the lost weight. The problem here is that you lost muscle and the body replaced the lost weight with fat. This is why yo-yo dieting destroys the metabolism and the BMR.

Turn Up the Furnace and You Turn Up the Heat

Current scientific evidence has established that muscle is the key to a healthy metabolism. As our body uses its sugar and fat as fuel to produce energy, heat is produced. A healthy metabolism produces 65 percent energy and 35 percent heat. A person with a slow metabolism conserves energy and does not produce adequate heat.

In the section on the ten biomarkers, biomarker ten (temperature regulation) is important to help set biological rhythms, and optimal muscle mass is essential to regulate body temperature. Biological rhythms are vital as we age. Scientists have demonstrated that proper body temperature is needed to activate certain alertness levels during the day, and as bedtime approaches, heat levels signal the brain to promote sleep. It has been well documented that if we do not get proper sleep, we cannot burn fat; and simply put, you don't lose weight. With the stress we face in today's world, our stress response is thrown off at a much younger age, and this affects the temperature, biological rhythms, and accelerates the biological age. Remember, a pound of muscle burns approximately ten calories while fat doesn't burn much at all. Losing muscle affects body heat, which is now recognized as an important issue in setting the stage for proper sleep patterns, and therefore, all other biological patterns.

Resistance Training and Optimal Health

Scientists have discovered that we lose eight ounces (1/2 pound) of muscle per year after the age of twenty, and it can be much more if the stress response is out of balance. They have also established that resistance training has been proven to be the most important activity to counteract the loss of muscle and its effect on health and aging.

Tufts University performed a study with a group of seventy-year-old individuals. In this study, participants performed resistance training twice a week. The results of the study showed that each individual increased their lean body mass and strength. When you increase muscle, you change the ten biomarkers, and invariably, you will restore and change your health. This change only comes through resistance training.

Health organizations, such as the American Heart Association and American College of Sports Medicine, have made aerobic exercise recommendations for nearly forty years. It hasn't been until recently that they started to advise people to do resistance exercises, such as weight training. Dr. Randy Braith and Dr. Kerry Stewart from the University of Florida showed that weight training had a positive effect on blood pressure by reducing the systolic and diastolic pressures by about three points (mmHg). Studies also show that people lose body fat when they train with weights, even without calorie restriction. It also contributes to the prevention and management of injury, slows bone and muscle loss, and prevents falls, and delays frailty in older adults. Weight training has significant health benefits independent of those provided by aerobic exercise.

Lilly's Story

Lilly is an eighty-seven-year-old client that was referred to me by her doctor. When I met Lilly, she was bedridden with a bilateral hip bursitis. It was very painful for her to move, let alone to get out of bed and walk. When she started the program, the first step was for me to get the circulation going. So we started with light stretching to get the muscles and blood flow moving. The next step came a couple of weeks later when we got her in a chair and started doing a few exercises and continued with the stretching. In each session, I would increase the amount of exercises, including new body parts. Then, with the aid of a cane, we started walking while increasing her resistance training. Within thirty days, we were able to perform a full workout and get rid of the cane altogether. Her strength was literally increasing each day, and along with the strength, an increase in her energy and a drastic change in her overall mood came. Today, Lilly trains at one of our centers using machines, dumbbells, and exercise bands, performing functional exercises that have literally given her a new lease on life. Lilly also uses the stationary bike as part of her aerobic training along with swimming. She is strong and fit and walks unassisted and is pain free.

After working for years, with a population with an average age of seventy years, I have learned some valuable lessons when it comes to wellness. One of the most important lessons I have learned is that you are never too old to get started and restore the body's health. I also learned that you are also never too sick to get started. The key that turns it all around is to manage the stress response, and the tool is proper exercise.

Traveling the world, I see many cultures, and the one thing they all have in common is STRESS! As I have devoted an entire book to the subject, I want to share one thing I have seen—stress makes us lazy and inactive. Obviously, if the stress response is off, we are more fatigued. For more than fifty years, scientists have known that factors such as high blood pressure, high cholesterol, and cigarette smoking increase the risk of coronary artery disease, heart attack, and stroke. In recent years, major risk factors have been expanded to include *physical inactivity, obesity, and diabetes*. There have been many changes in scientific research when it comes to measuring our optimal health. It has been discovered that more subtle changes in our metabolic health, such as blood vessel inflammation (silent inflammation) and blood clotting activity, are also involved in cardiovascular disease. Turkish researchers showed that middle-aged men who exercise regularly (three times per week) had *lower blood sugar, uric acid, triglycerides, higher levels of the good cholesterol (HDL), and enhanced function of the endothelial cells (cells lining the blood vessels)*. The answer is simple for maintaining optimal health, we have to preserve muscle and keep the biomarkers healthy. This is only accomplished with proper exercise and resistance training is a key element.

Resistance Training and Longevity

Muscle has a direct effect on our aging process, and it begins with losing half a pound of muscle after the age of twenty years. This rate accelerates after age forty-five because our hormones will begin to change. This condition is called sarcopenia, and it is the catabolic nature of aging. This loss of muscle is what accelerates our biological age and destroys our overall health and metabolism. When the stress response is not managed properly, this process accelerates. When we speak of longevity, it is not just about living longer; it is all about living well as we age.

Men will lose 20 percent of their muscle mass between the ages of forty and sixty. When we lose muscle, we gain fat, as our bodies are unable to use it adequately for fuel. British researchers found that smaller arm measurements are accompanied by increased waist sizes. They studied the death rate of 4,107 men age sixty through seventy-nine during a six-year period. Arm circumference and waist size were the two best predictors of death. Small arms increased the risk of death by 36 percent. The risk ballooned to 55 percent in men with waist circumferences above forty inches. Understand that when we lose muscle, we gain fat. So weight also doesn't matter as the researchers found that underweight men with a body mass index (BMI) of less than 18.5 (the proportion of weight and health), particularly those with larger waists, had the highest death rates. Most likely due to increased inflammation from where they stored their fat on their body.

The study was interesting because it again proves that the scale is a useless instrument for measuring health. The key to longevity and maintaining health at any age is the muscle-to-fat ratio and keeping the ten biomarkers at an optimal level. Lilly and Alan's stories are very common. It is not a miracle that this population improves so quickly. If the body is exposed to the right type of exercise, it will come back and restore its health, always. The bottom line is that resistance training is the longevity. We can eat right and do aerobic exercise, but if we are losing muscle, we will age and lose our health.

Lean Body Mass: resistance training routines and circuit training

Circuit training involves using a combination of resistance exercises done in a consecutive fashion that will work the muscles and the cardiovascular system together. With circuit training, you can create a workout where you are training the muscles and make it aerobic at the same time.

I have included some sample circuit routines for each cycle of health. But I must tell you that if you are not currently exercising or have not exercised for a long time, it is wise to hire a personal trainer to instruct you. If you have access to a BioFit Center, take advantage of it and work out with one of our health managers. The personal trainers who work at the Bill Cortright's BioFit Center are specially trained to help you practice your stress response program. The trainers at BioFit are referred to as health managers because they have advanced education on the program and special populations. If you do not have access to BioFit, you can take the book to your trainer and copy the routine so they can teach you. You can also have the trainer contact BioFit for more information at www.biofitprogram.com

There are several reasons why an investment in a personal trainer can make all the difference in the world.

1. The resistance movements need to be done with proper form to prevent injury and get the best results from the training. A personal

trainer will educate you in the beginning so you will know how each
exercise is set up and how it should feel.

2. You will have an appointment for the exercise session. It is simple.
    An appointment is a commitment. You have it in your schedule so
    you are more likely to stay with the program.

3. Remember in "Part Three: The Mind," we talked about creating
    habits by reprogramming the subconscious mind and the comfort
    zone? The key is to give the subconscious a new programming, and
    you must get through the first thirty days in order to create any type
    of new habit and lifestyle change. A good personal trainer will keep
    you motivated even when you don't feel like training. At times, they
    may have to drag you into the gym. After a while, you will find that
    when the habits are programmed and they will have to drag you out
    of the gym. I can tell you from personal experience that this is true;
    I cannot stand to miss an exercise session.

Working the Circuit

The way the circuit routines are set up is that three exercises make
one circuit. Start with the first exercise and do fifteen repetitions. Go to
the second, and then the third exercise, and perform the same number of
repetitions, fifteen. Once you finish the circuit, check your heart rate. If
your heart rate is below your ATR (from the calculations you did in the
previous chapter for your aerobic zone), then start with the first exercise
of the circuit and repeat the process. If your heart rate is high, let it come
back down to your zone before starting the next set. Let the heart rate drop
near your FBR before starting the next set of exercises. In the routines, I
have given you three sets of circuits. *Do not overexert yourself; if the heart
rate does not come down, then stop the session and call it a day.* Your exercise is
only as productive as how well you can recuperate. Too much or to intense,
you will throw off the stress response. Two to three times a week is enough
resistance training for most.

Overtraining: Too Much of a Good Thing

Simply put, overtraining is an imbalance between training and recovery.
When this happens, the stress response is completely thrown out of balance.
The consequences of this can be severe and include chronic fatigue, injury,
depressed immunity, and psychological depression. As we enter the second

cycle of health after thirty-five years, there is a fine line that exists between improving one's health and throwing off the stress response. The reason is simple; exercise is stress, and the body after age thirty-five years doesn't handle stress the same way it did just a few years earlier. Resistance training must be hard enough to stimulate muscle, but not too hard to throw off the stress response.

Symptoms of overtraining include the following:

- Elevated heart rate. Another good reason to always wear your heart monitor while training is it gives you automatic biofeedback on how the body is working.
- Chronic muscle and joint soreness and frequent injuries
- Frequent illnesses
- Psychological depression
- Abnormal behavior (like outbursts of anger).
- Constant cravings for sweets and carbohydrates
- Fatigue. You are yawning your way through the day, and even though you sleep enough hours, you still wake up tired.
- Most important, you will actually lose muscle and break down the ten biomarkers, accelerating your aging and increasing your body fat. Yes, you are working out and getting fatter. Just take a quick look around the gym; this is more common than you may think.

Stress-Response Exercise Recommendations

Before starting any exercise program, I strongly recommend that you get a physical and clearance from your doctor. If you are entering the second cycle of health and as young as thirty-five years and under a lot of stress, I now recommend a full physical along with a stress test. Every day at the BioFit Centers, we are seeing young people in there thirties with really bad lab tests and broken down biomarkers. If you are over forty years of age, you should get a yearly physical. That is a key to having a true wellness program; it is combining the program with your doctor with an attitude toward prevention.

BioFit Stretching and Resistance Training Sample workout

BioFit Exercise Guidelines:

* It is recommended that you do the stretching routine before or after every workout.
* Each workout is composed of four sets of three exercises each. You must perform the three exercises three times before moving on to the next set.
* If you are new to exercising and/or have never done resistance training before you may want to begin by doing one set (three exercises) per workout session and work yourself up to the four sets.
* You can practice these workouts two or three times per week.
* Always have a bottle of water with you while you exercise. Drink water after completing each set.
* If you have never done resistance training before start with 3, 5 or 8 pound dumbbells if you are a woman and 5, 8 or 10 to 12 pounds if you are a male.
* If you have practiced resistance training before, then you should use a weight that is challenging yet not too hard to work with. You will know if the weight is too heavy if you find that you struggle to complete the total of repetitions for each movement. If you have difficulty completing all your repetitions, lower the weight you are using.
* If you suffer from any medical or physical condition that may put you at risk if your resistance training exercises on your own, we strongly suggest that you seek the assistance of a professional Personal Trainer to guide you and assist you with these workouts.
* These workouts are recommendations based on what the training techniques practiced at the BioFit Center. It is always better to work out with a professional personal trainer when doing resistance training to avoid injury.
* The workouts shown here are only one workout per cycle of health. To get a custom—made workout plan for a month please visit our website: www.biofitprogram.com.
* The cycles of health are:

  Cycle I Age—25 to 35
  Cycle II Age 35 to 45
  Cycle III Age 45 to 55
  Cycle IV Age 55 and above

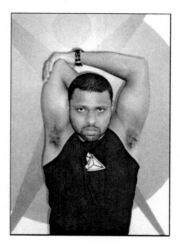

Tricep Stretch.

Pull Elbow behind your head holding on to it with your opposite hand.
Pull until you feel the muscle stretching. Repeat with other elbow. Hols for
15 seconds each time.
Do this one time per stretching routine

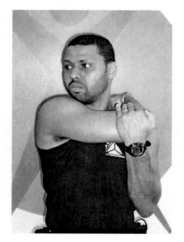

Posterior Shoulder Stretch.

Pull arm across Chest holding on to it with opposite hand until you feel the
muscle stretching. Turn your head away from pull. Hold for 15 seconds.
Repeat with other arm.
Do this one time per stretching routine

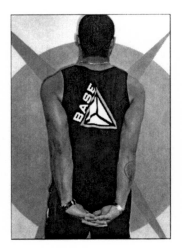

Behind Back Shoulder Stretch.

With finger interlaced behind your back, straighten aems and turn elbows
in until you feel the muscles stretch. Hold this for 15 seconds.
Do this one time per stretching routine.

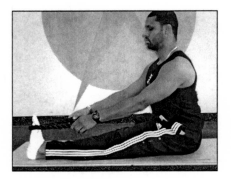

Lower Leg Stretch

Sitting on the floor with one leg straight out and the other one bent so that
the bottom of the foot touches the side of the knee, use a strap or small towel
to place on the ball of the stretched out foot, gently pull back until you feel
a stretch on the back muscles of your legs. Hold this for 30 seconds.
Do this one time per stretching routine

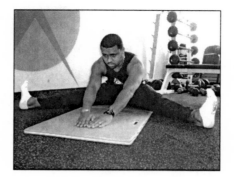

Groin Stretch

With legs apart, slide hands forward trying to keep your back as straight as possible until your feel the inner thigh muscles stretching. Hold for 20 seconds.
Do this one time per stretching routine

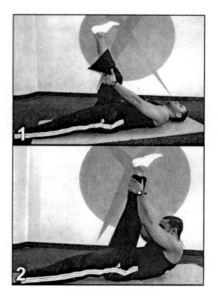

Hamstring leg raise stretch

Laying down on your back, with hands behind one knee, pull leg forward until stretch is felt in the back of the leg. Hold for 15 seconds. For a better stretch move hands up to the leg towards the ankle. Repeat with the other leg. Do this one time per stretching routine.

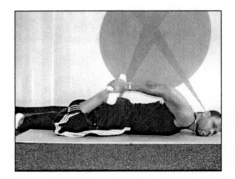

Front Thigh Stretch

Lying on your stomach with thighs together, gently pull ankle toward buttocks until you feel the stretch in the fron of your leg. Hold for 30 seconds. Repeat with other ankle.
Do this one time per stretching routine

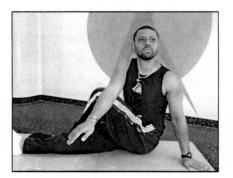

Oblique/Hip stretch

With left leg over right, bring right elbow (and arm) over left leg. Push the left leg across the body until you feel the stretch . Turn head over left shoulder. Hold for 30 seconds and repeat with the other side.
Do this one time per stretching routine

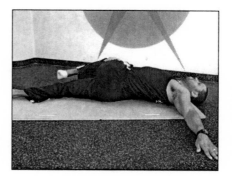

Laying down hip/Oblique sterch.

Laying on your back and keeping the shoulders flat on the floor, pull on bent leg toward the floor until you feel the stretch on your buttocks and lower back. Hold for 30 seconds and repeat with the other side.
Do this one time per stretching routine

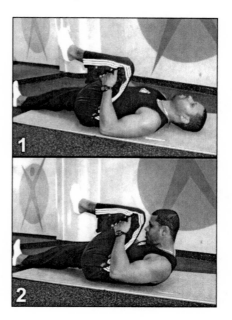

Lower back stretch

Laying on your back bring one knee to chest holding the back of the leg/ knee. Bring head to knee and hold for 30 seconds. Repeat this with the other knee. Do this one time per stretching routine

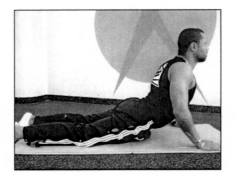

Abdoment and Chest Stretch.

Laying on your stomach push upper torso up with arms until stretch is felt
and Tilt head as far back as possible. Hold there for 45 seconds.
Do this one time per stretching routine

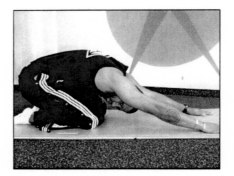

Upper Back Stretch

Sitting on your legs on the floor bring your torso forward. Slide hands
forward and buttocks back (on feet). Extend your arms on the floor as far
as they can go to get a better stretch on the back. Hols for 60 Seconds.
Do this one time per stretching routine

Cycle I—Age 25 and Younger to 35

Cycle of Health One: Below Twenty to Thirty-five Years Old

- Warm up for ten minutes with some light walking or any type of cardio exercise, not exceeding too much over your FBR.
- Follow the resistance routine three times per week on alternate days. Follow the recommendations from "Working the Circuit" with your personal heart rate.
- After the resistance training routines, spend ten minutes following the basic stretching routine.
- Do aerobic exercise, using either the interval routine outlined in the chapter on link three or fat-burning walking for thirty to forty minutes, three times a week. This can be done before or after your resistance training. To manage the stress response, it is better to do aerobic training on different days because it will give you an outlet. But because of individual time restraints, it is not wrong to do it on the same day as resistance exercise.

Note: Children under the age of twelve should consult a qualified personal trainer before doing any type of resistance training. At BioFit, we have many children that are doing resistance exercise as young as eight years, but the routines vary from child to child.

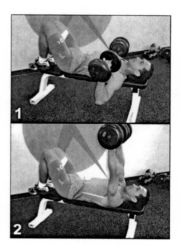

Chest Press

Laying on a bench with dumbbells in hand. Press hands and dumbbells up and down 12 times. Repeat this exercise 3 times.

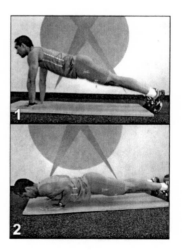

Push ups

Laying on your stomach place your hand at shoulder level against the floor. Push your body up by pressing the hands against the floor and keeping your entire torso as straight as possible. Push up and down 12 times. Repeat this exercise 3 times.

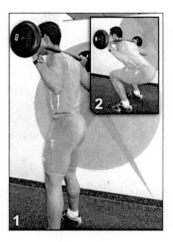

Squat with barbell.

Carefully rest a barbell across the back of shoulders and neck. Make sure you are holding it with both hands at all times. Once you are comfortable stand with your feet shoulder width apart. Bend your needs and bring your buttocks back and downwards as if you were going to sit on a chair. Lower your buttocks passed the knee height and back up. Do 12 squats. Repeat this exercise 3 times.

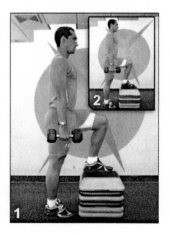

Step Ups

Using a step or a bench place on foot on top of it. Keeping your back straight and your head up, step up unto the the step or bench lifting your body weight with the leg on top of the bench or step. To better keep your balance you can do this movement next to a wall to hold on to. Do 20 step ups with each leg. Repeat this exercise 3 times on each leg.

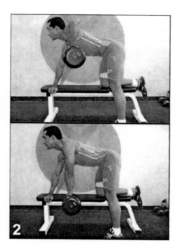

Bent over Row

Place one knee and and hand on a bench while the other leg remains stretched and the foot on the ground and the same side hand holds on to the dumbbell. Keeping your head up bring the dumbbell up by bending the elbow upward and then down by slowly allowing the arm to stretch downward. You should feel your back working while you lift the dumbbell. Do 12 rows. Repeat this exercise 3 times.

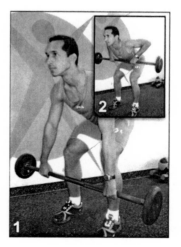

Bent over barbell Rows

Holding a barbell bent over forward and bend your kneed slightly. Hold the barbell with stretched arms and pull barbell up bending your elbows upward bringing the barbell to the abdomen. Do 12 rows. Repeat this exercise 3 times.

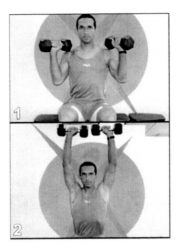

Shoulder Presses

With dumbbells in hand sit on a chair or the edge of a bench. Maintaining your back straight begin pressing your arms up above your head and then down keeping your torso strong and straight. Do 10 presses. Repeat this exercise 3 times.

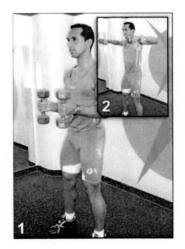

Shoulders lateral press

Standing with feet shoulder width apart and a straight back. Bent arms so that dumbbells are facing forward. Freeze arms in this position. Proceed to raise bent arms upward on each side as they remain bent. This puts all the pressure on the should muscles. Do 10 shoulder lateral presses. Repeat this exercise 3 times.

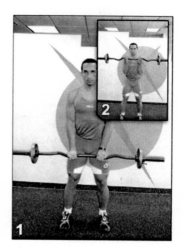

Bicep Curl with EZ barbell

Standing withy feet should width apart and a straight back. Curl arms up raising the EX barbell toward your neck and back down. Do 10 curls. Repeat this exercise 3 times.

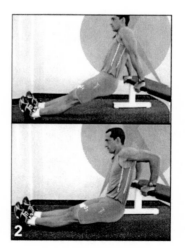

Dips

Start by sitting on the edge of a bench and placing your hands on each side of your body, holding on the bench. Slide your buttocks forward off the bench so that your arms are the only thing holding on to the bench. Keep your legs straight in front of you. Slowly bend your elbows bringing your buttocks down to the ground (while your legs remain straight) Then push up bringing your buttocks back up to the bench level and back down. Do 12 dips. Repeat this exercise 3 times.

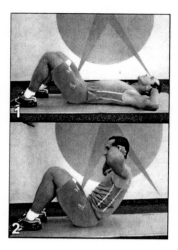

Abdominal crunch

Laying down on your back bend your knees so that your feet are flat on the ground. Place your hands behind your neck and head. Push your upper torso up while continuing to hold your head with your hands. Do 15 crunches. Repeat this exercise 3 times.

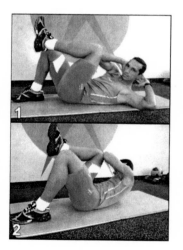

Alternating Crunches

Laying down on your back bend your knees so that your feet are flat on the ground. Place your hands behind your neck and head. Bring the right Elbow up and toward your left knee as you simultaneously raise the left knee toward the right elbow in a crunching motion. Do the same movement using the left elbow and the right knee. Do 20 crunches on each side alternating sides. Repeat this exercise 3 times.

Cycle II Age 35 - 45

Cycle of Health Two: Thirty-five to Forty-five Years Old

- Warm up for ten minutes with some light walking or any type of cardio, not exceeding too much over your FBR.
- Follow the resistance routine two to three times per week on alternating days. Follow the recommendations from "Working the Circuit" with your personal heart rate.
- After the resistance routine, spend ten minutes following the basic stretching routine.
- Do aerobic exercise using either the interval routine outlined in the chapter on "Link Three: Circulation" or fat-burning walking for forty to fifty minutes, three to four times per week. This can be done before or after your resistance training. To manage the stress response, it can be better to do aerobic training on different days because it will give you an outlet. But because of individual time restraints, it is not wrong to do it on the same day as resistance training.

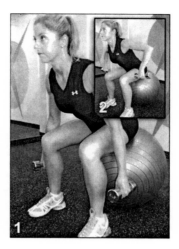

Row on Exercise Ball.

With dumbbells in hand sit on the exercise ball.
Bring your torso forward to rest on your thighs. Lift the dumbbells upward
as you bend your elbows up. Palms should be facing each other on each side
of the body. Do 15 rows. Repeat this exercise 3 times.

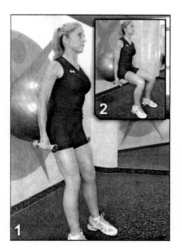

Squats against Exercise ball

With dumbbells in hand lean against the exercise ball, which you must place
against a steady wall.
Once your back in against the ball bend knees bringing your buttocks down
as if you were sitting on a chair. Do not allow your knees to pass your toes.
Do 15 squats. Repeat this movement 3 times.

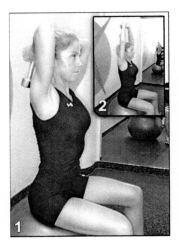

Tricep Overhead Extension

With dumbbell in hand sit on the exercise ball. Once sitted grab the dumbbell with both hands and plance above and behind your head carefully. With upper arms vertical, raise dumbbell by extending elbows. Keep feet flat and back straight.

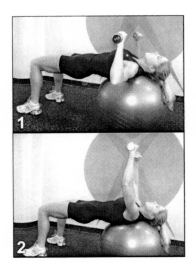

Chest Press on Exercise Ball

Begin by sitting on the ball with dumbbells in hand and slowly begin moving your feet away from the ball as your back leans on the in a supine position. Once in this position begin pressing up and down slowly.
Do 15 chest presses. Repeat this movement 3 times.

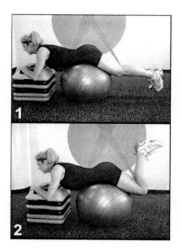

Hamstring Curl on exercise Ball

Find a steady surface to hold on to, position ball directly in front of it and lay on your stomach on the ball as you hold on to the steady surface. Place dumbbell between your feet and roll back until you are in a stretched position. Use your torso maintain your balance.
Begin flexing the knee to bring the dumbbell up with your feet.
Repeat this flexion 15 times. Repeat this movement 3 times.

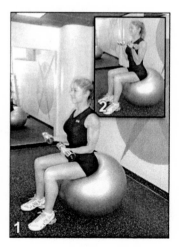

Bicep Curls on Exercise Ball

With dumbbells in hand, sit on the ball. Maintaining a straight back and strong torso begin curling the dumbbells upward and back down.

Do 15 bicep curls. Repeat this movement 3 times.

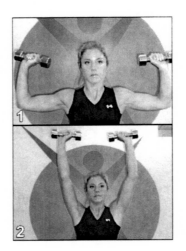

Shoulder Press on Ball

Seated on an exercise ball or a chair,
Keep back straight. Do 15 shoulder presses
Upwards maintaining the back straight.
Repeat this process 3 times.

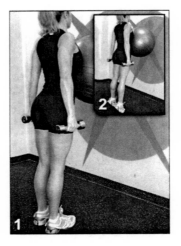

Calf raises against the wall

Lean on exercise ball and rise up on your toes
15 times. Repeat this process 3 times.

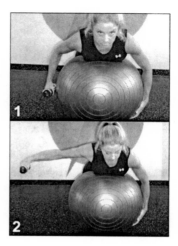

Shoulder, rear fly

Stomach on exercise ball, back straight, arms slightly bent.
Raise one dumbbell to shoulder level. Do 15 repetitions with each
Arm. Repeat this process 3 times.

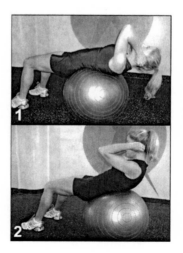

ABS - Crunch on ball

Hold hands together behind head to support your neck.
Do 15 repetitions then move to the next exercise.
Repeat this process 3 times.

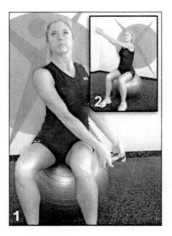

Wood chop on ball

Hold dumbbell with both hands, rotate trunk. By bringing both hands above opposite shoulder.
Keep pelvis stable on ball.
Do 15 repetitions then move to the next exercise.
Repeat this process 3 times.

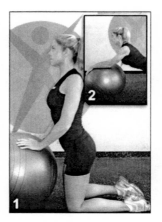

Exercise Ball Roll

Place hands on the ball keeping your back straight begin
To roll the ball forward. Progressively tense Ab muscles.
Be careful not to hyperextend lower back. Roll back to start position.
Do 15 repetitions then move to the next exercise.
Repeat this process 3 times.

Cycle III Age 45 - 55

Cycle of Health Three: Forty-five to Fifty-five Years Old

- Warm up for fifteen to twenty minutes with some light walking or any type of cardio, not exceeding too much over your FBR.
- Follow the resistance routine two times per week on alternating days. Follow the recommendations from "Working the Circuit" with your personal heart rate.
- After the resistance routine, spend fifteen minutes following the basic stretching routine.
- Do aerobic exercise, using either the interval routine outlined in the chapter on "Link Three: Circulation" or fat-burning walking for forty-five to sixty minutes, four to five times per week. I recommend doing intervals for thirty minutes and fat burning for the rest of the time. This combination really works well for this cycle of health. I also recommend for this cycle of health at least six hours of exercise minimum to manage the stress response. Two resistance and four aerobic sessions. Out of 168 hours in a week, we must give at least six to maintaining the machine.

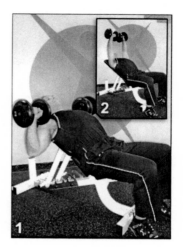

Incline chest press

With dumbbells in hand sit against the incline bench and begin pressing up and down. Do 12 presses. Repeat this exercise 3 times.

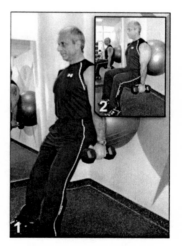

Legs Squat agains exercise Ball.

Carefully place the exercise on your middle back against the wall. With Dumbbells in hand. Bring your feet slightly forward as you lean on the ball. Lower your buttocks toward the ground in a sitting down motion, slightly leaning against the ball. Do 12 squats. Repeat this exercise 3 times.

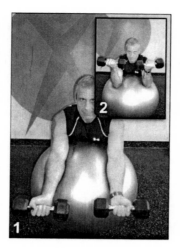

Bicep curls on Exercise ball.

Kneel over the exercise ball with dumbbells in hand. With elbows fully extended curl dumbbells up and down. Do 10 bicep curls. Repeat this exercise 3 times.

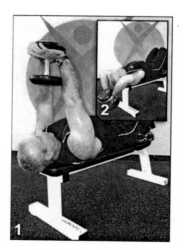

Pull over with dumbbell

Laying on back on a bench, hold dumbbell with both hands so that it hangs vertically from both of your hands. Hold your arms straight up in front of you, keep your legs bent and feet flat on the bench. Slowly bring dumbbell back over your head keeping your arms straight. Once you have completely extended your arms back bring them up slowly again to the starting position. Repeat entire movement. Do 12 pull overs. Repeat this exercise 3 times.

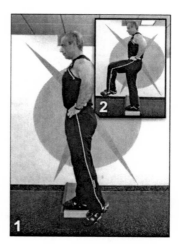

Hip/Knee Flexion.

With Left Foot on 10 inch step. Raise right hip at a right angle as you bend the knee up wards. Do 10 flexions on each side. Repeat this exercise 3 times.

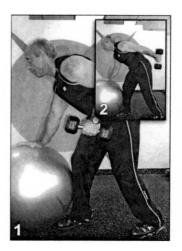

Tricep kickback on ball.

Stand with feet staggered, upper body supported by ball and upper arm parallel to floor. Raise the dumbbell by extending the elbow. Do the same with opposite arm. Do 10 kickbacks with each arm. Repeat this exercise 3 times.

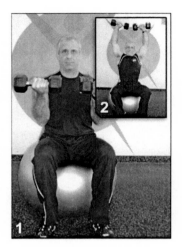

"Arnold" Shoulder Press.

Sitting on the exercise ball with dumbbells in hand keep your back straight. With hand facing upwards and elbows bent bring arms up sideways creating a circle from top to bottom. Movement should end above your heads, dumbbells together and palms facing downward. Bring arms back down following the circular motion. Do 12 Arnolds. Repeat this exercise 3 times.

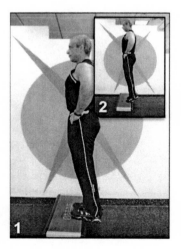

Calf Raises.

Place toes on board or step, heels on the floor, knees slightly bent. Rise up on toes as high as possible. Do 15 calf raises. Repeat this exercise 3 times.

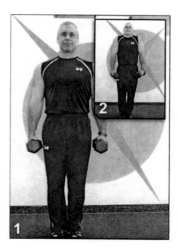

Trap shrug

Knees slightly bent, dumbbells in hand and body and torso straight shrug your shoulders upward and downward. Do 12 shrugs. Repeat this exercise 3 times.

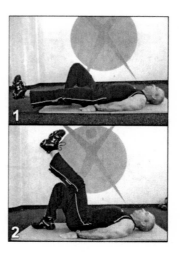

Single leg raise

Laying on your back, one leg bent and other leg straight on the mat. Raise the straight leg up toward ceiling, keep hips on mat. Lower it slowly back down. Do 10 leg raises. Repeat this exercise 3 times.

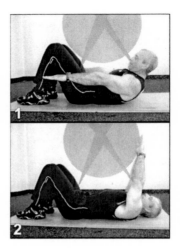

Straight arm crunch

Laying on your back, knees bent, feet on the floor. Straighten arms in front of you and crunch your torso upward bringing your arms down to the side of your body. Bring torso back down and arms back up and in front of you as you lay your back on the floor again. Do 10 cunches. Repeat this exercise 3 times.

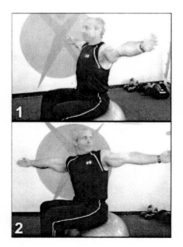

Twist.

Sit up straight , with legs presses together, feet flexed. Reach arms to the sides palms facing forward, inhale and as you exhale twist torso to one side maintaining arms straight. Bring torso back to initial position. Again inhale and exhale while you twist torso to the opposite side. Do 10 twists on each side. Repeat this exercise 3 times.

Cycle IV Age 55 and above

Cycle of Health Four: Fifty-five Years and Older

- Warm up twenty minutes with some light walking or any type of cardio, not exceeding too much over you FBR.
- Do the basic stretching routine after the warm up to prepare the body for the resistance training.
- Follow the resistance routine two times per week on alternate days. Follow the recommendations from "Working the Circuit" with your personal heart rate. For this cycle of health, I highly recommend that you invest in a good personal trainer to help and monitor your exercise sessions. *For clients over sixty-five years of age* at the BioFit Centers, we will train them in three different areas—flexibility and strength, balance, and cognition. At Cortright, we specialize in this population.
- After completing the resistance training, I recommend to repeat the basic stretching for another five to ten minutes. These exercises are so important as we age for circulation and preventing injury.
- Do the aerobics, maintaining your heart rate between your FBR and heart rate ten points higher. Basically, it is walking. I do not recommend intervals until you reach a good level of conditioning (usually two months of consistent training) or you have supervision from an exercise professional. The main key here is to exercise to build up oxygen and manage the stress response to guarantee healthful aging.

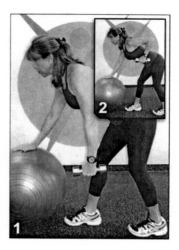

Row on Exercise Ball

With Feet staggered and one arm supported on the ball pull dumbbell to side of chest, keeping elbow close to the body. Keep back straight. Do 10 rows with each arm. Repeat this exercise 3 times.

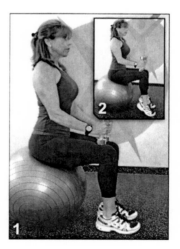

Sitting calf raises.

Sitting on the exercise ball with dumbbells in hand pace them on your thigh above the knee. Raise up heels pressing toes down. Do 15 raises. Repeat this exercise 3 times.

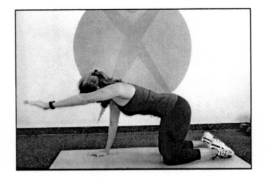

Upper body extension.

On your knees and hands on the floor or mat raise right arm in front without arching neck or back. Be sure to keep back flat. Do the same alternating with the left hand. Do 10 body extensions. Repeat this exercise 3 times.

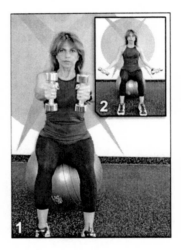

Sitting Fly.

Sitting on the exercise ball with dumbbells in hand. Extend arms to each side of the body, palm facing front. Bring both arms up in front of the body towards midline so that palms face each other. Bring them back down. Do 12 sitting flies. Repeat this exercise 3 times.

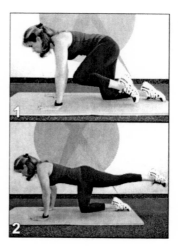

Kick backs

On hands and knees bring one leg in by bending the knee inward, keeping your back straight. Then extend leg out and up. Bring leg back down and in. Do 12 kick backs with each leg. Repeat this exercise 3 times.

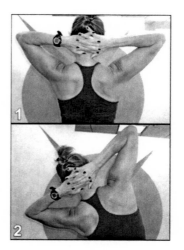

Spinal Mobilization

Place hands interlocked behind the head, tip right elbow up as you bring left elbow down. Keep the movement sideways and avoid tilting forward. Do 3 spinal mobilization exercises for each side. Repeat this exercise 3 times.

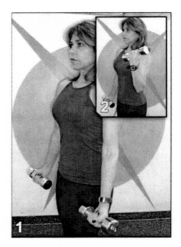

Bicep Curl

Standing up, feet shoulder width apart. Dumbbells in hand and palms in. Curl one arm up as you turn arm to have palm face up at the top of the curl. Do the same with the other arm. Do 20 curls. Repeat this exercise 3 times.

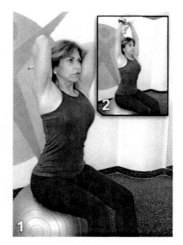

Tricep Overhead Extension

With dumbbell in hand sit on the exercise ball. Once sitted grab the dumbbell with both hands and plance above and behind your head carefully. With upper arms vertical, raise dumbbell by extending elbows. Keep feet flat and back straight. Repeat this movement 3 times.

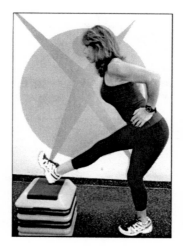

Hip/Knee stretch

Place left foot on stool, chair or bench. Slowly lean forward, keeping back straight until you feel the stretch in the back of the leg. Do the same with the right leg. Do 3 stretches per side. Repeat this movement 3 times.

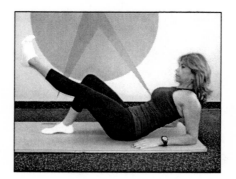

Hip/Knee straight leg raise

Resting forearms on the floor or mat and keeping on leg bent, keep the other leg straight. Raise the straight leg up keeping foot flexed. Do 10 raises per leg. Repeat this movement 3 times.

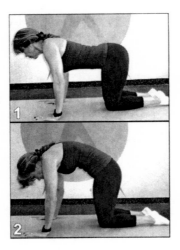

Cat Stretch

On your hands and knees, tuck chin in and tighten stomach while arching back. Do 5 cat stretches. Repeat this movement 3 times.

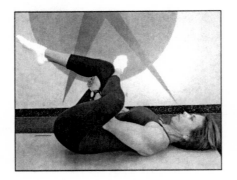

Piriformis stretch.

Laying on your back cross leg, right on top. Gently pull other knee toward chest until stretch is felt in buttocks/hip and top of leg areas. Do the same placing the left leg on top. Hold each stretch for 10 seconds. Do 3 stretches per side. Repeat this movement 3 times.

Benefits of Resistance Training

In 1976, Dr. Kenneth Cooper made the statement "you can live without big muscles, but you can't live without a healthy heart." Back then, many exercise experts thought that people who ran less than twenty miles per week were doing nothing to enhance their health and longevity. Considering that the heart is a muscle, and muscle is the key biomarker for health, Cooper and most other experts have modified their views of resistance training. In 2000, the American Heart Association officially recognized the contributions of resistance training to cardiovascular health. Resistance training is a vital component when it comes to cardiovascular health, weight management, and preventing disabilities and falls. Resistance training is as important as aerobic exercise for all aspects of longevity and optimal health. Here are a few of the benefits of resistance training:

1. Keeps the biomarkers at optimal levels a key component for aging
2. Improves posture and maintains optimal joint health
3. Rehabilitates old injuries
4. Increases bone density
5. Tones and shapes the body
6. Increases your metabolism and BMR
7. Increases aerobic capacity and energy levels
8. Maintains and improves balance
9. Enhances the cardiovascular system
10. Balances many hormones in the body including the stress response

Measuring Your Progress

The stress-response diet program is geared toward restoring the health of the body by managing the stress response and maintaining healthy biomarkers. When the biomarkers are at a healthy level, you produce optimal energy and lower the biological age. The key to healthy biomarkers is the muscle-to-fat ratios (3:1 for women, 5:1 for men).

Muscle is the key to optimal health, weight management, and longevity. The less muscle you have, the higher your body fat will be and the lower your muscle-to-fat ratios. This is the challenge of using the scale as a tool to measure your progress on the program. For instance, most anorexic people are actually "skinny fat people." Anorexics can have a body fat percentage as high as 40 percent, even though they are deadly thin. The reason for this is because they have lost so much muscle that their body composition is very high in fat.

The challenge with the scale is that you can actually lower your body fat levels and gain weight. If you weigh two hundred pounds and are 25 percent body fat, you have fifty pounds of fat. If you gain 10 pounds of muscle, you will have 210 pounds body weight and have 23.8 percent of body fat. Plus, in 95 percent of all clients, when the muscle increases, the fat goes down due to the body's increased calorie burning ability brought about by having increased the body's lean body mass. So please, do not worry about what the scale says; in fact, it is better not to use the scale as a measurement tool. Use your body composition and your body measurements as a marker of your progress. The way your clothes fit is a great measurement tool also; buy yourself some great clothing that is a size smaller than you are currently wearing. Try this clothing on every week until it fits perfectly, then go down the next size. This exercise always works without fail.

Taking Measurements

Below, you will find the body measurements you should take before you begin the stress-response diet program. A wonderful trick that will help you is to take the measurements, and then add up all the numbers. Every week, retake the measurements and keep track of your measurement sum. This way, you can track your total number of your measurements as if it is an overall score. This is much easier for you to see your overall progress.

Another great way to track progress is to get a body composition analysis from a reputable health club or your doctor. This will be able to give you an accurate measurement on the weight you are losing, whether it is lean body mass or fat.

Five Important Measurements for Women

1. Upper abdominals: two inches above the waist
2. Lower abdominals: one inch below the belly button
3. Waist: measure it at rest. It is important that you do this measurement relaxed; don't hold it in.
4. Hips: around the bikini line.
5. Thighs: around the widest part of the thigh.

Add all five measurements for your total score. Keep track of this number weekly or biweekly.

Five Important Measurements for Men

1. Chest: at nipple level.
2. Upper arms: center of the biceps.
3. Waist: measure it at rest. It is important that you do this measurement relaxed; don't hold it in.
4. Hips: around the widest part.
5. Thighs: around the widest part.

Final Word on Bio-Links Three and Four, Stress Response and Exercise

No one can argue with the fact that the stress levels in today's world are sky-high. During the time that I am writing this, the world is going through an economic recession, and many people are really starting to do a life review. We have lived through three decades of total excess. We have supersized value meals that we can pick up without getting out of the car, and we can easily consume thousands of calories before our main entrée ever arrives to the table. To top things off, we live a sedentary lifestyle, logging many hours every day sitting in front of a computer, and then rushing home so we can sit some more and watch our favorite television programs. All of this throws the stress response out of balance. No wonder we are all so tired and have cravings to eat more and more food, and no matter how much we eat, we are still hungry, storing more fat after each bloated meal.

The answer is to balance the stress response, and it is impossible to do so without proper exercise. We need aerobic exercise for increased oxygen and to utilize the body's ability to use fat for energy. We have been taught that we have to push hard, and that is just wrong. When doing aerobic exercise for fat loss, it doesn't matter how many calories you burn; what matters is what type of calories you burn. Your goal is to burn off excess fat. We need monitored exercise that helps us to balance stress, not increase it. We need to work in our zones three to five days per week.

We have also been programmed to believe that aerobic exercise is all we need to be healthy. The truth is resistance training is your only true answer for longevity and permanently increasing your metabolism. With stress comes muscle loss, and less muscle means a slower metabolism; a slower metabolism means more fat storage, which equals poor health. Resistance training can also enhance structural integrity of joints and connective tissue, which means you have an increased ability to stay active no matter what your age is. By following the right type of resistance training routine, you will increase the body's ability to utilize calories, balance hormones (including the stress response), and lower your biological age. All you need is two to three resistance sessions per week.

If time is a factor, use the stress-response exercise circuits in your aerobic zone, and you get the benefits of both resistance and aerobic exercise in an hour's time. But you must do it.

We would like to thank: Felipe Carvalho, Belinda Benn, Carlota Lozano de Del Rio and Luis Carlos Pena for posing in the exercise pictures for this book.

Chapter Twenty

Bio-Link Five: Junk Night
The importance of taking one
day off from your SR Diet

"The best cure for an off day is a day off"
—*Frank Tyger*

Summer of 1984
Junk Night Was Discovered

During the summer of 1984, I discovered something that changed my life and training forever. I was preparing for my first bodybuilding championship. I was serving in the United States Navy at the time and had become known as somewhat of a weight-loss expert but was really having trouble with my own program.

I had been struggling to make my competition weight. For twelve weeks, I had been eating as little as six hundred calories per day and training two to three times a day, totaling six to eight hours of exercise (I really had no idea what I was doing back then.) With one week to go, I had not lost a single pound in a month, and I had to drop another six pounds to make my weight class. Needless to say, I was getting very worried. With a little more than a week before the competition, I was called to travel out of town to take care of a family emergency. When I was on my way back to the base from this emergency trip, something happened that changed my dieting life drastically.

I was on the road, and it was late at night when I became very tired. I was so dieted down that I could barely keep my head up, so I decided to stop for a cup of coffee. I pulled up to a twenty-four-hour restaurant off the highway. I sat down and leaned on the counter on the verge of exhaustion. While I ordered my cup of coffee, I spotted a blueberry muffin in a pastry container on the corner of the counter. I had already consumed my allotted calories of six hundred (as I write this, I cannot believe how insane I was—six hundred calories?) for the day, but I couldn't help telling myself, *One muffin won't hurt. I will just do extra cardio tomorrow. After all, I still have two hundred miles to drive, and I really could use the energy.* Anyone who has ever been on any type of diet knows the voice I am talking about.

Boy, what a mistake! After eating the muffin, I triggered a binge response, and my body went into survival mode. I simply could not stop eating. I am not kidding when I say it was an overwhelming urge to eat. I literally felt possessed, like it was life or death. I ordered six muffins to go and ate two more before I even reached the car. Once I was back on the road, the other four muffins were consumed like there was a vacuum, but I wasn't even close to being satisfied. I pulled up to a gas station and loaded my car with all types of junk food, and basically, I didn't care about the competition any longer. The gas station was not the last stop, about thirty miles down the road, I found a restaurant that served pizza. I had not had pizza for months (my favorite food), and I ate a large pizza by myself. I kept eating until I finally began to feel sick. I was forced to pull over and get a hotel room for the night; there was no way I could travel any farther. If you have ever been on a binge (most dieters have been), you feel very helpless because you literally cannot stop eating. I was so depressed. After months of the hard work I had put into preparing for the competition, with days left, I had blown it. I had failed not only myself, but also all my friends and family who were supporting me. It was quite a low point in my life.

I arrived early that morning back to base. I was so tired and still feeling the effects of my food hangover. I was afraid of the damage I had done to my body after the binging episode from the night before. When I took off my clothes and looked into the mirror, I couldn't believe what I saw. In bodybuilding terms, I was *ripped.* I could see perfect muscle definition, and I was so vascular (my veins were showing). When I stepped on the scale, I almost fell over. I was six pounds lighter than the week before. I had eaten probably tens of thousands of calories, and I now stood in front of the mirror looking better than ever. Not only did I look ready for competition but I had also lost the weight I needed to lose to be able to compete in the show. I went on to win that show, and that is when bio-link five, junk night, was born.

During that trip, before my first contest and thanks to my feast blowout, I had discovered firsthand the final link of my program. For the last twenty-five years, I have had a day off; and during this time, I have incorporated this ritual in all my client's programs around the world. Junk night makes the program workable for a lifetime of health. How does cheating actually make the stress-response program work? The two reasons why junk night is so important are its psychological and physiological effects.

Psychological Benefits of Junk Night

Let's say I have just given you the greatest program ever put together for health management. But there is one catch, and that is you can never again eat cheesecake. And let's say cheesecake is one of your favorite foods of all times. It is simple; you can attain perfect health if you never again consume cheesecake. What is the only thing you are going to be thinking about? You are not going to be thinking about the stress response, biomarkers, bio-links, or anything of the sort, you will only be thinking, "I better go out and get some cheesecake before I start this program."

The stress-response diet is a lifestyle program that will restore your health, help you reach your goals, and most importantly, help you maintain your health for a lifetime. Yes, you will lose weight (fat), but the great news is you will not gain it back. In the stress-response diet program, you can literally have your cake and eat it too. For six days you follow your program; and on the seventh, have anything that you desire. Understand that this works psychologically because the mind rejects negative instructions. As we discussed in "Part Three: The Mind," most people focus on what they don't want. We literally are not wired to diet. Saying you are not going to eat this or that just causes you to want that food even more. With the junk night, we can say we will have that cheesecake on Saturday after you just went out for pizza. Junk night makes the program real, so you can still celebrate special occasions without guilt; in fact, you get to celebrate every week that you are managing your health and the stress response with a day off.

Once I implemented the junk night into the program, that night off once a week where I could eat the foods I wanted and was craving, something began to happen to my body. First of all, I was constantly energized and never felt depressed. I know now the reason I felt so great was because I was keeping the stress-response balanced by not letting my body fall into starvation mode (famine). The second thing was I no longer craved junk food and came to the realization that there was no such thing as bad food. I was able to eat whatever I wanted once a week, and I always felt satisfied. Many times, I don't eat any junk at all, just more carbohydrates and more calories. Junk night doesn't have to be junk food; but it does have to break the pattern of your diet. Over the last twenty-five years, junk night has gone to junk day or even junk weekend for some people (more on this later in "Junk Night Guidelines").

Junk night makes your program real; it is a great psychological tool, but the stress-response diet program is not psychological, it is scientific. Let's take a look at how cheating helps the body lose weight.

Physiological Benefits of Junk Night

In "Bio-Link One: Meals," you learned that in order to produce fat loss and increase fat burning, you had to manage the stress response and you must lower your fat set point. Let's make this explanation as simple as possible. If you have gotten this far in the book, you have learned one main lesson about the human body, "the body is built to survive." The body's main survival fuel is fat; any time the body is out of balance, it will store fat. So let's say I give you a perfect diet of 1,800 calories, and you follow this perfect diet every day. Our body is built to survive, so it knows that it is only receiving energy (food) in the amount of 1,800 calories. So the body will lower its metabolism so it will only burn 1,800 calories. Remember, to lose weight, we have to have the body burn more calories than it consumes. Now the only way you can burn more fat is to lower the calories. The challenge with that is our survival mechanism. If you eat fewer calories than your basal metabolic rate, the signal to the body is that there is not enough food (famine), and once again, the body's survival mechanism kicks in. Once the body perceives that there is not enough food, it will cause the stress response to become imbalanced. The body will release more cortisol so it can break down more muscle so the body can produce energy. Because the body is in famine, it cannot burn fat. This is when we get insatiable cravings and low energy levels, and we will usually binge. Once again, the ending of another diet. This process explains why diets don't work. Even those who have had weight-loss surgeries will gain the weight back if they don't change their lifestyle and manage the stress response.

Why is cheating on your diet exactly what the body ordered? Let's go back to the same scenario. You are consuming 1,800 calories per day. But this time, you are following your diet perfectly for six days. On the seventh day, you take you junk night and eat whatever you want, consuming many calories over your regular daily intake. The body will perceive this increase in calories and will literally raise its metabolism to get rid of the extra calories. This is increasing your metabolism, and the next day, you go back on your regular menu with a faster metabolism. I have found over the years that junk night is as important as the other four links to keep the body healthy and burning fat. This day off keeps the body in a state of feast so the signal to the body is that it does not need stored fat, and thus, lowers your fat set point; helping you keep the weight off.

Junk Night and the Leptin Hormone

In chapter 14, we discussed hormones and fat loss. Scientists have identified more than 250 factors that control body fat, appetite, satiety, fat storage, and fat breakdown. These include neurotransmitters in the brain, hormones produced by various endocrine organs, and chemicals released in the gut. As we have discussed, when you cut down on the food you eat, your metabolism slows; and when this happens, the appetite will increase. The reverse will happen when you eat more than you need for resting and exercise metabolism. *This is why junk night is so important physiologically, because it balances important hormones that control appetite.* We discussed many of these hormones in chapter 14, such as leptin, PYY, CCK, grehlin, and neuropeptide Y. Scientists that have been testing these different hormones are trying to figure what is best for people to be able to lose weight. Most scientist will agree that the leptin hormone is one of the key players. Leptin depresses the appetite and increases the metabolic rate. In fact, in one study, leptin caused a 20 percent weight loss in obese rats within a few weeks. Unfortunately, when leptin was given to humans, they didn't get the same results. The reason, as we discussed in chapter 14, is that most overweight people are leptin resistant. In other words, they have leptin; but their brain is resistant so the signal to the body is low leptin, causing the body to slow its metabolism and increase hunger for survival. Improved leptin metabolism is the key to a healthy fat-burning metabolism. Junk night plays a role by overfeeding the body for one day to balance leptin.

Junk Night Guidelines

Junk night is a simple link, but a very important one. It is important physiologically and psychologically. I don't have a lot of rules when it comes to this link, but here are a few notes of caution. First, if you have any medical conditions such as high blood pressure, insulin resistance, metabolic syndrome, and especially diabetes, DO NOT OVERDO IT. Please be sensible with your junk night. I have learned many tricks over the years that I will share with you. Here are some suggested guidelines:

1. Try to pick one day a week (usually Friday, Saturday, or Sunday). I have found that Saturday works best for me. Many clients use Sunday, but when I do that I don't have as much energy on Monday. Experiment to find out what is best for you. You may also take a junk night on a different day for special occasions.
2. If you are on a phase one menu, your junk night is one full meal during the day. You can have it at lunch or dinner, eat until you are satisfied.
3. If you are on a phase two or three, your junk night is actually a junk day. This is a free day. Some clients have tried to make this a twenty-four-hour period. In other words, they start at night and take it to the next day, ending with lunch. For some clients (usually those under health cycle one), this is not a problem. But for those that are older, it doesn't work very well. There is too much change in the chemistry. Try to keep this Junk Day simple, have something you have been craving for breakfast, a little something special for lunch and dinner. Don't go crazy with junk food or high sugar deserts, you might make yourself sick because your body has cleansed from excess sugar during the week.
4. If you feel that the junk night makes you want to binge, try the following: Control your junk night by eliminating desserts and sticking to more starches and only have one "junk night" meal that day. A good rule to follow is to throw away any leftover food from junk night. This will eliminate any temptation that will keep you from returning to your menu once junk night is over.
5. A great exercise to help compulsive overeaters, such as myself, is to make a list during the week of the foods you want to consume on junk night. For instance, if on Wednesday, you see someone eating

peanut M&M's, and you really want to have some, write it down on your junk night list. This little exercise of keeping a JN list helps to reprogram the subconscious mind. The mind is satisfied to know that it will get that food on your junk night. Remember, when you manage the stress response, you will not have physical cravings. So it becomes easy to fool the mind.

6. Another trick I use is to have a very hearty breakfast the day after the junk night. The day after, you will actually find yourself hungry in the morning because the metabolism is in high gear. I have a large breakfast the day after JN. It will consist of my regular breakfast carbohydrate intake and much more protein and fat (huge omelet with bacon, cheese, and two slices of bread with peanut butter). You get the idea. By doing this, you will not feel like overeating throughout the day.

7. The following day after junk night, it is great to do some fat-burning aerobic exercise for thirty to forty minutes. I have found that this helps to balance the stress response quickly so you will not have cravings. It is also a great psychological tool to get back on track without problems.

8. Have fun and do not feel guilty! Eating the things you like and may crave is not going to hurt once a week. As we discussed, the chemistry of the diet is important; in fact, it is key in managing the stress response. Remember that the fat-burning hormones need to receive a signal of feast to balance out. Junk night is as important as exercise, so enjoy.

I have now followed the stress-response diet program for over twenty-eight years. I can tell you, without this link, there is no way I would have kept off one hundred plus pounds for this long. This link allows me to be free and to be able to celebrate special occasions without upsetting the balance of my lifestyle program. During my diet years, while I was attempting to lose weight on every diet imaginable, the most difficult thing was the cravings for my favorite foods. With junk night every week, I get to have everything and anything I crave. This is a special link in the stress-response diet program that makes the program real for anyone who follows it. It was years later before I learned the science behind why junk night worked, but I can tell you this link is the savior for thousands of people following the program. Please enjoy!

Final Thoughts

It has become painfully obvious that over the last quarter of a century, obesity in America is the number one health issue in this country. According to the Centers for Disease Control and Prevention, 64 percent of American adults age twenty years and above are obese or overweight. Being obese puts you at risk for heart disease, diabetes, strokes, etc. In England, at St. Thomas's Hospital, researchers found that an increase in a person's BMI (body mass index) causes oxidative stress and increases aging at a molecular level. When you are overweight, the biomarkers are broken down so your body will have less oxygen and will not be able to burn fat properly. When this happens, the body no longer handles stress throwing off the stress response, causing more breakdown of the biomarkers. It is literally a viscous cycle.

The simple solution is to manage the stress response and restore the health in the body. All five bio-links are key to accomplishing this. Understanding how the mind works is essential for you to create new habits and to balance the stress response.

What I have shared with you in this book is a lifetime of research. It works! I promise you, after as little as two weeks, you will notice the difference. My mission with this book is to create a worldwide movement of wellness; so please, as you succeed, pass it on. Thank you.

Conclusion

Congratulations on getting started on your new path with the Stress Response Diet and lifestyle program.

In the journey I have traveled seeking answers for what it takes to lose weight and keep it off, I came to the understanding that I had to have three things to succeed.

1. I had to understand how my body worked. I also needed to know why the programs I did in the past failed. I realized that it wasn't my fault; the programs were doomed because they went against our built-in survival mechanism. Education is very important when you try to make lifestyle changes.
2. I had to understand how to create new habits. How the Mind plays a key role when it comes to our body and overall health. Self-sabotage comes from subconscious programming that you had no control

over. Understanding the mind and its testing periods allows you to program your comfort zone for a lifetime of success.

3. I had to understand that the key to health and weight loss is consistency. Follow the Five Bio Links and you cannot fail. Everyone needs a map and with this book I have laid out exactly what you need. I know it works because not only have I worked with thousands of people but I have managed to keep the weight off for 28 years. I tell everyone, if I can do it anyone can.

I am here to support you. Please contact me at our BioFit on-line program at *www.biofitprogram.com* or you can twitter me directly @BillCortright. I wish you all health, well-being and prosperity.

He who has health has hope; and he who has hope has everything.
—Arabic Proverb

Appendix A

The Stress Response Diet Panels
Understanding your blood test results

I have used blood tests for years to help me in the process of creating balanced lifestyle programs. Blood Laboratory tests are a magnificent tool to evaluate not only the health status of clients but also how their bodies process foods and manage stress. Over the years I have realized that many of the values used for certain blood test results are ruled by reference values that are not entirely accurate. This inaccurate range reference confuses people. Many already feel "sick" or are symptomatic yet show "normal" ranges in certain tests. This is a recurring issue especially with certain hormone levels and thyroid levels. At Bill Cortright's BioFit Centers we use a slightly different "normal" range reference which we find to be much more accurate. We also use specific and unique blood test panels to see how the body is working so that we can create the right program for the individual. For us, Blood tests are one third of the equation; we use them in combination with the BioFit cardio metabolic stress test and all the subjective data the client gives us on how they are feeling during the evaluation process. Here is a short explanation of the blood tests panels we use so you can interpret your own blood work and some supplement recommendations. **Note: the blood test panels BioFit recommend are not intended to diagnose illness or to give medical advice. Always consult your physician before taking any type of supplements.**

Blood Fats: Cholesterol is a fat-like substance in the blood, which is responsible for hormone balance, and if the wrong cholesterol is elevated it can be a major risk factor for heart disease. I use the BioFit Omega 3 Fish oil and CLA Fat metabolizer to balance the ratio between good and bad cholesterol. If triglycerides are high I recommend our BioFit Fat Burner/ Sugar Blocker Formula.

- **Total Cholesterol:** High cholesterol in the blood is a major risk factor for heart disease. What many people don't understand is that cholesterol in itself is not bad. Our bodies need a certain amount of cholesterol to maintain health. I don't worry about the overall cholesterol number as much as the breakdown of the different types of cholesterol. Most doctors will want the **overall cholesterol at less than 200.**
- **LDL Cholesterol (low density lipoprotein):** This is considered the "bad cholesterol" because this cholesterol deposits in the arteries when levels are elevated. **Optimal LDL levels are below 100.** Values greater than 160 are considered high risk.
- **HDL Cholesterol (high density lipoprotein):** This is considered the "good cholesterol" because it protects against heart disease by removing excess cholesterol deposited in the arteries. You could have very high HDL, which may bring your overall count to above 200. You would not be at risk for heart disease if this were the case. **Optimal HDL levels are above 50.**
- **Triglycerides:** This is fat in the blood created when the body does not process carbohydrates well. I went into detail on these fats in the book. High triglycerides can be associated with heart disease and pancreatitis, especially when they reach levels over 500. Elevated triglycerides lead to lower HDL levels. **Optimal triglyceride levels are below 150 (I strive to get them below 100).**
- **VLDL Cholesterol (very low density lipoproteins):** This is also bad cholesterol. VLDL is elevated when triglycerides are high. If you bring down the triglycerides you will bring down the VLDL. VLDL is another carrier of fat in the blood. **Optimal VLDL levels are 20 or lower.**

Glucose: This is a measure of the sugar level in the blood. High values can be associated with metabolic syndrome or diabetes. I have seen elevated glucose levels in people on the Atkins Diet when they are eating virtually no carbohydrates. This is because you can have higher than normal glucose levels when the Stress Response is out of balance. I will recommend the BioFit Insulin Resistance Formula to my clients to naturally balance this. **Optimal Glucose levels are 60-95.**

Complete Blood Count (CBC): The CBC can tell us a few things. Here is what I look at to design a lifestyle program.

- **White Blood Count (WBC):** This is the number of white blood cells in a sample of blood. High WBC can be a sign of an infection. WBC is also increased in certain types of leukemia. Low WBC can be a sign of bone marrow disease or an enlarged spleen. Even though I don't order test to diagnose illness sometimes abnormal results signal red flags. When this happens we recommend to the client to mention the findings to their physician in their next visit. Sometimes the results show an elevated WBC, which could be a sign of increased inflammation in the body. A low WBC, I have found, is associated with unmanaged stress. That is why many people get sick when they are under too much stress due to a repressed immune system. **Optimal values are the reference values of the test.**

- **Hemoglobin (Hgb):** The hemoglobin is the amount of oxygen carrying protein contained within the red blood cells. Hemoglobin transports oxygen from the lungs to the rest of the body where it releases the oxygen for cell use. Low oxygen equals low fat burning which equals low energy and bad health. Low hemoglobin may suggest anemia. When the hemoglobin is toward the low side I increase the B-Vitamins (BioFit Stress Management Formula). If it's really low we recommend they see their Doctor. **Optimal values are the reference values of the test.**

- **Platelet Count (PLT):** Platelets are cells that work to prevent bleeding when a cut or tissue injury occurs. High values can cause increased clotting of the blood and may be at an increase risk of a stroke. When the platelet count leans toward the high end it may mean that the client has increased inflammation. When platelets are elevated I increase healthy fats in the clients diet and limit omega-6-fatty acids to balance the diet. In these cases I also recommend BioFit Omega-3 Fish Oil supplement. When the platelets are on the low end of the reference values you should not take an Omega-3 supplement, because this can cause further blood thinning and inhibit the body's ability to clot properly. I also never recommend that a client take an Omega-3 supplement if they are on blood thinner medications. **Optimal values are the low to mid reference ranges 180-250.**

Thyroid: The majority of my client's average age is around fifty-years-old. By working with this age group I have found that many of them have lower than optimal thyroid function, especially women after menopause. The ovaries have thyroid receptors and the thyroid gland has ovarian receptors. So when a woman goes through menopause it can also change the way the thyroid functions. As we discussed in the book, an imbalance of thyroid hormone can throw off every metabolic function of the body. When measuring the thyroid I look at **thyroid stimulating hormone (TSH), thyroxine (T4) and triiodothyronine (T3). I also request the free T4 and the free T3 because high levels of estrogen such as birth control can give an elevated T4 reading. The free T3 and T4 measure the portion of the thyroid hormone that is free and not bound to carrier proteins.**

- **TSH:** This protein hormone is secreted by the pituitary gland and regulates the thyroid gland. If TSH levels are high it suggests that you have a slow thyroid or hypothyroid. If TSH levels are low it suggests that you have a fast thyroid or hyperthyroid. **Optimal Values are 0.3-3. Many labs reference ranges are just too high, some as high as 6. If your TSH is on the high end and you have symptoms of a hypothyroid please contact an endocrinologist to study the options for possible treatment. It will change your life.**
- **Free T4:** Measures the T4 hormone that is not bound to carrier proteins in the body. The T4 free for the body to use. T4 is produced in the thyroid gland. **Optimal values are above .7-2.0.**
- **Free T3:** Measures the T3 hormone that is not bound to carrier proteins in the body. The T3 free for the body to use. Your body produces both T4 and T3. T4 is converted to T3 in your liver or kidneys. T3 is five times more active for the body than T4. This is important because its key for your metabolic health and most doctors don't order it on the initial screening. You can have a perfect TSH and T4 and the T4 is not converting to T3 adequately you will have symptoms of a slow or hypothyroid. When I see the T3 is low and the TSH and T4 are normal I will give the client the BioFit Daily Formula and selenium to aid in the conversion. If the client is symptomatic of hypothyroid I send them to a good doctor. **Optimal values are 3 or higher.**

Hormones: Throughout the Stress Response Diet we have talked about balance, especially hormone balance. The Stress Response is about balancing

Cortisol and Insulin. There are also sex hormones, metabolic hormones and regulatory hormones. These are some of the labs we use for hormones:

- **Cortisol:** The adrenal glands produce cortisol 24 hours a day with a regular diurnal variation. Cortisol output is the highest within the first hours of waking and declines steadily throughout the day, with its lowest levels during sleep. Cortisol is one of the key players in the Stress Response Diet as its function is essential for balancing blood sugar, weight control, sleep, mood and the stress response. If your levels are too high or too low the Stress Response is off. I will usually give the client BioFit Corti-Lean Formula and BioFit Stress Management Formula for B-Vitamins. **Optimal values A.M. 12-18. Note: At this time I am starting to learn more about Saliva Testing and the information states that it is much more accurate because it measures cortisol throughout the day. Also I never do a PM cortisol because I am not diagnosing illness. If there is an abnormal A.M. test we send the client to the MD.**

- **Insulin:** Insulin is the hormone that regulates your blood sugar levels. If Insulin becomes unresponsive or resistant (cannot remove the blood sugar), your blood sugar will rise and you will not be able to burn fat. When this happens you will develop metabolic syndrome or Type 2 diabetes. High insulin can be associated with hormone imbalance in woman by increasing testosterone and lowering estrogen levels. Increased insulin will also increase your body fat especially the dangerous fat stored around the middle. Low insulin levels can be associated with hypo-glycemia or low blood sugar. I have found that most people with low insulin have an inbalanced stress response. With low insulin the cells cannot get the nutrients that needs and the body breaks down. For elevated insulin I give the clients BioFit Insulin Resistance Formula. If they have insulin resistance or really elevated insulin I send them to the MD. For low insulin I give the client extra protein. Especially between lunch and dinner around 3-4 pm when the Stress Response is the highest. **Optimum fasting values 5-8. Anything over 15 needs a phase one menu, because you will not burn fat until it comes down.**

- **DHEA-S:** DHEA is a hormone made by your adrenal glands. DHEA production declines with age starting in the mid to late twenties. By age seventy we will make one fourth of the amount we did in our younger years. DHEA has been shown to help the body deal with stress. DHEA is important in balancing the Stress Response, as it is a counter balance to Cortisol. Low DHEA higher cortisol and vice versa. It supports the immune system and converts into our sex hormones including estrogen, progesterone and testosterone. I have found especially in men that DHEA will drop before testosterone will. Thus keep DHEA balanced and the other hormones usually will follow suit. DHEA is a hormone and should not be taken unless you have low levels. If your DHEA levels are too you can throw the rest of the hormones off. At Bill Cortright's BioFit Centers we don't recommend supplementing with DHEA unless you have been tested and have low levels. We also recommend retesting after six weeks to make sure the levels are good and not too high. BioFit DHEA is pharmaceutical grade giving the best supplement available to raise the blood levels to healthy values. **Optimum values above 300 for men and above 250 for woman.**

- **Estradiol:** This is the most common type of estrogen measured in woman. The levels vary with age and whether or not they are having normal menstrual cycles. Estradiol is the main estrogen a woman's body produces before menopause and is the estrogen they lose at menopause. Men also produce estradiol and will have increased levels as they age due to the decrease in testosterone. By age 55 men will have higher levels of estradiol than women of the same age. The BioFit Woman's Hormone support formula can give natural support to a woman and relieve hot flashes. For replacement you must contact your physician. **Optimum values are the reference ranges for pre-menopause woman and above 60 in post menopause. In men below 25.**

- **Progesterone:** This is one of the sex hormones and is produced in the ovaries before menopause. After menopause, some progesterone is made in the adrenal glands. Progesterone is a precursor to most other steroid hormones, including cortisol and testosterone. In men progesterone is produced in adrenal and testicular tissue. Progesterone in men is important because it inhibits the conversion of testosterone to dihydrotestosterone (DHT), which is a stimulant of prostate cell growth. For progesterone replacement you should consult your doctor. Men should also consider this when using hormone replacement with their doctors. **Optimum values are the reference ranges for pre-menopause woman and above 1, ideally 2 for post-menopause woman. In men less than 1.**

- **Testosterone:** Levels of testosterone decline in men as they enter the Second Cycle of Health about age 35. The age-related decrease in testosterone is called andropause (male menopause), which is linked to muscle loss, decreased Biomarkers, depression, declining sexual performance and reduced interest in sex. Woman with low testosterone will have similar symptoms including the reduced interest in sex. The key in measuring testosterone is determining the free or available amount of testosterone. Most men's total testosterone will remain rather leveled within normal values, even as they age. The biologically available testosterone (free testosterone) will drop by 50% in middle-aged men between the ages of 30-60. In woman testosterone is made in the ovaries and adrenal glands. As a woman ages the ovaries will produce less testosterone. The BioFit Men's Hormone Support formula works wonders on increasing a male's free testosterone naturally. I have seen a 30-50% increase in the blood tests in as little as 30 days. **Optimal values for men are Total 500-800 and Free above 15. For woman Total reference ranges and Free above 1.**

Hemoglobin A1C: This measures the amount of glucose chemically attached to your red blood cells. Since blood cells live about 3 months this test can tell you what the average blood sugar has been for the last 6-8 weeks. We use this test as reference with those with metabolic syndrome and type 2 diabetes. We also get a base line number on everyone after the fourth cycle of health. This allows us to do yearly comparisons on the client. The BioFit Fat Burner & Sugar Blocker along with Insulin Resistance Formula can help the client to lower this. **Optimal value is 5.5 or under but must be below 6.0.**

Electrolytes: These are important tests if you are taking certain medication for hypertension. This test measures your potassium, sodium, chloride and CO_2 levels.

- **Potassium:** Is controlled very carefully by the kidneys. It is important for the proper functioning of the nerves and muscles, particularly the heart. When we see clients especially those in the third and forth cycle of health, which are experiencing a lot of muscle cramps we will check their electrolytes. It is important for anyone taking a diuretic or heart pill to take a good multi-vitamin/mineral everyday.

Newer evidence suggests that dietary potassium may play a key role in decreasing high blood pressure. It is not generally recommended to take a potassium supplement alone; it is better to take it with a dose of vitamins and minerals. The BioFit menu is also naturally high in potassium. The BioFit Ultra Complete Multi Vitamin Multi Mineral is a complete one a day with a perfect balance of vitamins and minerals. **Optimal value is the lab reference ranges. Any value outside the expected range, high or low, requires a medical evaluation.**

- **Sodium:** As with potassium is also regulated by the kidneys and the adrenal glands. Most Americans take in way too much sodium in their diet that can lead to elevated sodium and high blood pressure. Approximately ten percent of people with high blood pressure are sensitive to dietary salt (or sodium). A reduction of sodium in the diet helps lower the blood pressure in all people with hypertension. **Optimal value is the lab reference.**

- **Chloride:** Plays a key role in helping maintain a normal balance of fluids in the body. Elevated chloride is usually seen in episodes of diarrhea and certain kidney diseases. Chloride is normally lost in urine, sweat and stomach secretions. Decreased chloride can be caused from heavy sweating, vomiting and adrenal and kidney disease. **Optimal value is the lab reference.**

- **Bicarbonate (or total CO2):** Reflects the acid status of your blood. Low CO2 levels can be to increased acidity of your diet or from uncontrolled diabetes, kidney disease, and metabolic disorders. **Optimal value is the lab reference.**

Waste Products: When creating a menu to manage the Stress Response one of the main components of the menu is protein. As we have discussed, protein is a key nutrient to balance and manage the Stress Response. In fact protein is an important nutrient that is key to the health of every cell in your body. The challenge is that some people do not metabolize or process protein well. Protein is an acid-forming food, so if you take in too much (the body can only simulate approximately 25-30 grams in one meal) or don't metabolize it you will create a more acidic blood. The key is creating an alkaline balance by eating a lot of vegetables.

The following tests are important to know if you have to monitor your protein intake.

- **Blood Urea Nitrogen (BUN):** This is a waste product produced in the liver and excreted by the kidneys. Elevated values may mean that the kidneys are not working as well as they should. BUN is affected by high protein diets and/or strenuous exercise, which also raise its levels. Elevated values will mean that you will have to consume less protein per serving. **Optimal value is the lab reference.**
- **Creatinine:** This is a waste product largely from muscle breakdown. When there is an elevated value along with an elevated BUN level, this may indicate problems with the kidneys. As with BUN you need to watch the amount of protein per serving. What I do with clients in this situation is start them on the menu and then measure the BUN/Creatinine along with the Ten Biomarkers (ELG test) and make adjustments to the diet accordingly. **Optimal value is the lab reference.**
- **Uric Acid:** is normally excreted in urine. Elevated values are associated with gout, arthritis and kidney problems. The diet plays a key role here. When elevated you should avoid high purine foods, limit meat, chicken, fish to 6 ounces, and avoid alcohol especially beer. There are other protein choices I usually recommend such as dairy, eggs or whey protein supplement. Increased water intake at least three liters a day is recommended. **Optimal value is the lab reference.**

Enzymes: AST, ALT, GGT, LDH and Alkaline Phosphatase are abbreviations for proteins called enzymes. These enzymes help all the chemical activities within the cells to take place. Injury to the cells releases these enzymes into the blood. These enzymes are found in muscles, liver and the heart. Elevated values are caused by a number of diseases such as alcohol disease. I have also seen elevated levels in clients with a fatty liver or taking cholesterol lowering medications.

- **Alkaline phosphatase (AP):** AP can be elevated in many types of liver disease. AP is an enzyme produced in the bile ducts and sinusoidal membranes of the liver. Increased AP can be caused by bile duct blockage, damage to the bones or liver. **Optimal value is the lab reference.**
- **GGT:** This is often elevated in those who use excessive alcohol or other liver toxic substances to excess. Elevated GGT along with

elevated AP, suggest bile duct disease. Elevated GGT can also be caused by fatty liver disease. **Optimal value is the lab reference.**

- **LDH:** This enzyme is present in all cells in the body. LDH is in many tissues, especially the heart, liver, kidney, skeletal muscle, brain, blood cells and lungs. Anything, which damages cells, including strenuous exercise will raise LDH in the blood. **Optimal value is the lab reference.**

- **ALT:** This test was previously called SGPT and is more specific for liver damage. It is generally increased in situations where there is damage to liver cell membranes. ALT is also elevated with a fatty liver, some drugs/medications, alcohol and liver and bile duct disease. Many times I see this elevated in clients with high triglycerides. After a couple of months on the menu these values many times return to normal. **Optimal value is the lab reference.**

- **AST:** This test was previously called SGOT. AST is a mitochondrial enzyme that is also present in the heart, muscle, kidneys and brain. AST can be elevated with liver inflammation due to a fatty liver or some types of medications or illness. **Optimal value is the lab reference.**

- **Bilirubin:** Is a major breakdown product that results from the destruction of old red blood cells. Bilirubin is a pigment removed from the blood by the liver. Low values are of no concern. If slightly elevated above expected ranges, but with all other enzymes (LDH, ALT, AST, GGT) within expected values, it is probably a condition known as Gilberts syndrome (GS). GS is a hereditary disease that causes harmless jaundice and is not significant. **Optimal value is the lab reference.**

- **CPK:** This is an enzyme, which is very useful for diagnosing diseases of the heart and skeletal muscle. CPK is the enzyme that is first elevated after a heart attack, especially the first 3-4 hours. If CPK is high in the absence of heart muscle injury, this can be a strong indication of skeletal muscle disease. CPK can be elevated in diseases such as "Progressive Muscular Dystrophy" where there is a continuing loss of muscle. Also CPK can be elevated if you had a hard workout the day before the test was done. **Optimal value is the lab reference.**

Proteins: As we have discussed throughout the book, proteins are the building blocks of all cells and the body's tissues. Proteins also play a major role in maintaining the delicate acid/alkaline balance in the blood. The major measured serum proteins are divided into two groups, albumin and globulins. A typical blood panel will provide four different measurements, total protein, albumin, globulin and the albumin/globulin ratio.

- **Total Protein:** This measurement represents the sum of albumin and globulins, it is more important to know which protein (albumin or globulin) is high or low than the value of the total protein. When the total protein is elevated it can be due to chronic infection, liver dysfunction, disease (Rheumatoid arthritis, systemic lupus), dehydration, alcoholism. Total protein can be decreased due to malnutrition, liver disease, kidney disease, and diarrhea. **Optimal value is 6.5-8.0 g/100ml.**
- **Albumin:** Is synthesized by the liver using dietary protein. Albumin levels are a very strong predictor of health. Increased albumin levels can be from dehydration, poor protein utilization, glucocorticoid excess (from increased cortisol or cortisone medications). Decreased albumin levels can be caused by dehydration, hypothyroidism, malnutrition, liver dysfunction and diarrhea. I find this very valuable when setting up a lifestyle program, as it is an important window into the individual's health. **Optimal values are 4.0-4.8 g/100ml.**
- **Globulin:** These are proteins that include gamma globulins (antibodies) and a variety of enzymes and carrier/transport proteins. These are important for fighting disease. Increased globulin values can be from chronic infection, liver disease, and Rheumatoid Arthritis and kidney disease. Decreased globulin values can be caused by liver dysfunction and kidney disease. **Optimal values are 2.8-3.2 g/dL.**
- **A/G Ratio (Albumin/Globulin Ratio):** The proper albumin to globulin ratio is 2:1. An increased A/G Ratio can be caused by hypothyroidism, high protein/high carbohydrate diet, low globulin, glucocorticoid excess (increased cortisol or cortisone medications). Decreased A/G Ratio can be caused by liver dysfunction. **Optimal value is 1.7.**

Cardiac Risk Factors: This is a group of tests along with the lipid profile that can help determine if you have an increased chance of developing cardiovascular disease. These are important test when creating a lifestyle program as they can determine balancing factors in the diet and supplements for the body.

- **High Sensitivity C Reactive Protein (hs-CRP):** This is the key marker for inflammation and a key test I use in a majority of the clients after entering the second cycle of health. In the past this test was used to assess inflammation in response to infection. Today hs-CRP is used in predicting vascular disease, heart attack or stroke. When the hs-CRP is elevated that is a sign of inflammation. This can be caused by an imbalanced diet of the omega3 and omega 6 fatty acids. Elevation has also been shown with stress, fatty liver, hypothyroid, diabetes and metabolic syndrome. What has been shown to lower the hs-CRP are statin drugs, weight loss, exercise, niacin, and quitting smoking. When I have a client with elevated inflammation I will make sure the fats are balanced in their diet by decreasing the omega-6-fatty acids and increasing the omega-3 fatty acids. I have had great results with supplementing the BioFit fish oil supplements from 1-3 grams per day. **Optimal value is below 1.0.**
- **Homocysteine:** This is an amino acid that is normally found in small amounts in the blood. Higher levels of homocysteine are associated with increased risk of heart attack and other vascular diseases. Elevated homocysteine levels may be due to a deficiency of folic acid or vitamin B12, due to heredity, older age, kidney disease, or certain medications. It seems that men will usually have higher levels. To reduce homocysteine you must change your diet to include more green leafy vegetables and consume fortified grain products or cereals. The BioFit Stress Management Formula is built to take care of this with its extra folic acid and combinations of B vitamins. I recommend clients with increased homocysteine to take the BioFit Stress Management Formula in the morning and the BioFit Ultra Complete Multi Vitamin at night. **Optimal values are 4-15, but if you have been diagnosed with cardiovascular disease you should try to keep it below 10.**
- **Lipoprotein (a) or Lp (a):** This is an important test in the prevention of cardiovascular disease. Lp(a) is a lipoprotein consisting of an LDL (bad cholesterol) molecule with another protein (Apolipoprotein (a)) attached to it. Lp(a) is similar to LDL cholesterol, but **does not respond to typical strategies that lower the LDL cholesterol such as diet, exercise or cholesterol lowering medications.** The level of Lp(a) appears to be genetically determined and not easily altered. Clients with elevated Lp(a) I am much more aggressive in

making sure the other factors such as lipids, triglycerides, glucose and insulin levels are in optimal range. I usually recommend the BioFit Fish Oil up to 3 grams a day to push the HDL (good cholesterol) higher. I also recommend the BioFit Metabolizer CLA, Stress Management Formula, Insulin Resistance Formula (If they have elevated triglycerides or sugar) and Ultra Complete Multi Vitamin. **Optimal value is the lab reference.**

Appendix B

Stress Response Diet & Lifestyle Program Suggested Wellness Blood Test Panels

Basic Stress Response Panel:

- Total Cholesterol
- LDL
- HDL
- Triglycerides
- Fasting Glucose
- CBC (Complete Blood Count)
- TSH (Thyroid)
- Free T-4
- Free T-3
- Fasting Insulin
- Cortisol AM

Second Cycle of Health (35-45)

- **Basic Stress Response Panel**
- Hs-CRP
- Hemoglobin A1C
- Homocysteine
- Urinalysis
- PSA free and total (men over 40)
- Lipoprotein (a)

Third Cycle of Health (45-55)

- **Basic Stress Response Panel**
- **Second Cycle of Health Panel**
- Total Testosterone (Both Men and Women)
- Free Testosterone (Both Men and Women)
- Liver function
- Bun/Creatinine
- Estradiol (Both Men and Women)
- Progesterone (Women)
- DHEA-S

Fourth Cycle of Health (55 and older)

- **Basic Stress Response Panel**
- **Second Cycle of Health Panel**
- **Third Cycle of Health Panel**
- Electrolytes
- Folic acid
- Uric acid

These are panels we use at the BioFit Center as a screening tool to design personalized BioFit Programs. The medications you take and the state of your health at the moment of the test will influence the results each time. We do not use these blood tests results to diagnose any specific condition, only certified and qualified physicians can do so.

We intereprete the blood tests to find markers which will help us design the personalized BioFit plan the person needs and the information drawn from these panels is used to define what type of nutrition, exercise and supplement regimen is best for you as an individual. **The Stress Response Diet and lifestyle program is not intended to diagnose illness or replace medical advice. For medical treatment or illness screening you should always consult with your doctor.**

Appendix C

Stress Response Diet and Lifestyle Program
BioFit Supplement Formulas

1. **Antioxidant Formula (Co-Q10):** CoQ10 is involved in all oxygen utilizing metabolic reactions (aerobic) within the body and helps muscle cells convert fat and carbohydrates for energy. Research supports the use of CoQ10 in controlling blood pressure and preventing heart disease by reducing LDL (bad) cholesterol. As an antioxidant, CoQ10 is important because it regenerates the antioxidant power of vitamins C and E. This keeps the free radical damage down and helps with slowing the aging process. Anyone taking a statin medication to lower their cholesterol must supplement their diet with CoQ10. Statin medications decrease the body's production of CoQ10. I **Recommend that anyone with high cholesterol or in the second cycle of health and above take 50-200 mg of Antioxidant Formula (Co-Q10) per day.**

2. **Insulin Resistance Formula:** This is a formula I created to help people with metabolic syndrome; those individuals like myself who don't process carbohydrates well. The main ingredient is chromium. Chromium is essential for helping the body to maintain optimal insulin performance which is a key hormone in the Stress Response. In the Insulin Resistance Formula I use two type of chromium, **chromium polynicotinate and chromium picolinate.** This helps to significantly reduce carbohydrate cravings. Newer research has found that chromium also helps to blunt the catabolic hormone cortisol, which is the other key hormone in the Stress Response. The other two ingredients that make up this formula are. **Alpha-Lipoic-Acid (ALA) and Biotin.** ALA has been shown to reduce the amount of insulin released, from the pancreas into the bloodstream,

by helping the cells to uptake the sugar thus lowering the insulin response when you eat carbohydrates. Biotin is a B vitamin that is needed for the formation of fatty acids and glucose, which are essential for the production of energy. Biotin helps with the metabolism of carbohydrates, fats and proteins. This supplement is **recommended for anyone with elevated sugar or triglycerides. As we age our bodies will have more trouble processing carbohydrates so Insulin Resistant Formula can help. Take 1-2 caps with a meal containing carbohydrates. I do not recommend IRF if you are taking blood sugar lowering medications, and as always talk to your doctor before taking any supplements.**

3. **Omega Max Fish Oil:** Fish oil contains the omega-3 fatty acids eicosapentaenoic acid (EPA) and docosahexaenoic acid (DHA), which offers numerous health and performance benefits. These essential fats have been shown to reduce the risk of heart disease and stroke, boost immune and brain function, increase joint health and help the body to burn fat. I **Recommend it for anyone diagnosed with increase inflammation and those with high LDL (bad) and low HDL (good) cholesterol. I also recommend it to everyone who is the third cycle of health and older. If you are taking a blood thinner medication you must talk to your doctor before taking this supplement. Take 1-3 grams with food twice to three times a day.**

4. **Metabolizer CLA:** This fatty acid is found in meats and dairy products. CLA has had many studies on its effectiveness, as a fat burning supplement but it is so much more. A double blind, randomized, placebo-controlled study, published in the December 2000 issue of the Journal of Nutrition found that CLA not only reduces fat but also preserves muscle tissue. The studies showed that CLA was found to increase metabolic rate, decreases abdominal fat, enhances muscle growth, and lowers cholesterol and triglycerides. I have found this to be true over the years especially with clients with elevated triglycerides. I **Recommend Metabolizer CLA Formula for anyone diagnosed with metabolic syndrome, elevated cholesterol and triglycerides and those wanting to lose abdominal fat. Take 1-3 grams daily with meals.**

5. **Stress Management Formula:** When we get stressed out one of the first symptoms we become aware of is that we get tired more easily and more frequently. The combinations of the B vitamins are critical for producing energy as well as the metabolism of amino acids, carbohydrates and fat. The B complex also offers other benefits such as proper nerve and immune function. The Stress Management Formula also contains

vitamin C and extra folic acid. The vitamin C is a powerful antioxidant that protects immune system cells from damage and allows them to work more efficiently. The Folic Acid is a B vitamin also known as folate and is critical for the production and maintenance of new cells such as muscle cells. Folate also plays an important role in the conversion of arginine to nitric oxide (NO). This is so important because Nitric Oxide relaxes and dialates blood vessels to prevent heart disease and strokes. The Stress Management Formula has twice as much folate as other B supplements for this reason. I **Recommend it for anyone with elevated homocysteine levels, metabolic syndrome, cardiovascular disease and diabetes. I also recommend it for anyone in the second cycle of health and above. Take one tab in the morning with breakfast.**

6. **Fat Metabolizing Formula:** I created this formula to give the body maximum potential of burning fat for energy without any negative side effects of stimulates. It contains the following ingredients:

- **Forskolin:** Is the active compound in the herb coleus forskohlii, a member of the mint family, forskolin enhances fat loss by activating the enzyme adenylate cyclase. This leads to a cascade of events including activation of the hormone-sensitive lipoprotein lipase, which allows fat stored in the fat cells to be broken down so it can be used as fuel. A study from the University of Kansas (Lawrence) found that over-weight men who took forskolin for 12 weeks lost considerable more body fat than the placebo group. Forskolin has also been shown to play a major role in a variety of important cellular functions including, inhibiting histamine release, relaxing muscles, increasing thyroid function and most important increasing fat burning activity.

- **L-Carnitine:** Carnitine is derived from an amino acid and is found in nearly all cells of the body. Carnitine plays a critical role in energy production. It transports fat into the cells mitochondria so it can be burned to produce energy. It can be found in avocados, dairy products and red meats (especially lamb and beef).

- **Green Tea:** Green tea contains compounds called catechins, including epigallocatechin gallate (EGCG), the primary active ingredient responsible for the tea's fat burning effects. Green tea does contain some caffeine, which is also great for fat burning; its major fat burning effect comes from the EGCG. EGCG has the ability to inhibit an enzyme that breaks down norepinephrine, the neurotransmitter involved in regulating metabolic rate and fat burning. Green tea also provides numerous other health benefits everything from relieving headaches to lowering cholesterol.

- **Quercetin:** This is the most abundant of the favanoids. Quercetin has many health promoting effects, including improvement of cardiovascular health and reducing the risk for cancer. Quercetin has anti-inflammatory and anti-allergic effects. All these activities are caused by the strong antioxidant action of quercetin.

- **5-Hydroxytryptophane (5-HTP):** This modified amino acid is what the essential amino tryptophan is converted to before it forms serotonin and melatonin in the body. 5-HTP has been shown to increase serotonin, which can decrease the cravings for sweets and carbohydrates (essential for the Stress Response) and melatonin which can help relax you before bed. In a study from the University of Rome, subjects taking 5-HTP ate fewer calories per day and lost an average of 11 pounds in 12 weeks, while a placebo group had difficulty limiting caloric intake and lost only 2 pounds in the same period. **Fat Metabolizing formula is recommended for anyone with elevated cholesterol, triglycerides and blood sugar. It is a safe and effective way to help the body to use its fat stores for energy. Since it is a complete formula 1-2 capsule a day with a meal is all that is needed.**

7. **Fat Burner and Sugar Blocker Formula:** This is a specialty formula I created for glucose management, appetite control, and to help reduce food cravings. I have added chromium picolinate for insulin management to allow the body to burn fat more efficiently. I have also added two different types of fiber for glucose management and to drastically reduce the appetite while lowering cholesterol. The Fat Burner/ Sugar Blocker also has three ingredients that work together to regulate the blood sugar levels. These are the main ingredients:

- **Chromium Picolinate:** This is important for helping the body to maintain optimal insulin performance a key hormone in the Stress Response.

- **Glucomannan (Amorphophallus Konjac Root):** This is the main ingredient in the Fat Burner/Sugar Blocker. Glucomannan is a water-soluble dietary fiber that is derived from the Asian konjac root. When mixed with water, it expands up to 50 times its original volume.

This aspect gives Glucomannan tremendous benefits: It curbs hunger and the appetite by filling the stomach and giving a feeling of "fullness", causing you to consume less calories. Glucomannan also delays stomach emptying, slowing the digestion and absorption of all nutrients, including carbohydrates, which leads to more stable blood sugar levels and prevents major spikes in insulin. This all aids in keeping the Stress Response in balance. The other great affect of glucomannan is that it binds to bile acids and carries them out of the body (through evacuation). This prompts the body to convert more cholesterol into bile acids and results in lower levels of blood cholesterol and other fats, which helps prevent weight gain.

- **Psyllium Husk:** This is one of the more popular fibers and is the main ingredient in most fiber supplements. The reason psyllium has been recognized as an excellent means of getting more dietary fiber into a persons diet is due to its high fiber count in comparison to other grains. For example Oat Bran is a good source of fiber, it has about 5 grams of fiber per third cup as supposed to psyllium husk, which has 71 grams of fiber per the same third cup.

- **Bitter Melon, Fenugreek and Mulberry:** All three of these ingredients play a role in regulating the blood sugar levels and managing the Stress Response. Bitter melon is great for glycemic control of the diet. Fenugreek fiber content plays a role in its ability to moderate metabolism of glucose in the digestive track. This is great for glucose control and lowering triglycerides. Mulberry has been shown to delay the absorption of carbohydrates and prevents sugar spikes, which can throw off the insulin hormone. These ingredients combined work toward optimal glucose management. **The Fat Burner/Sugar Blocker Formula is recommended to anyone with elevated cholesterol, triglycerides and blood sugar. It is great to decrease over eating and cravings for carbohydrates. Anyone looking to increase fiber in his or her diet and lose weight should add this formula to their daily diet. For optimal results take 1-2 caps 30 minutes before a meal with 8oz of water. Do not take Fish Oil or CLA along with this supplement, as it designed to remove fat from the body (good and bad). If using FB/SB take the fat-soluble supplements between meals.**

8. **Women's Hormone Support Formula:** This formula is a great support formula for women who are postmenopausal. It can help with hot flashes

and more important with bone density by slowing bone loss. This is also a great formula for women who suffer from menstrual disorders such as dysmenorrhea (painful menstrual cramps).

- **Ipriflavone:** This is a synthetic isoflavone, which is used to inhibit bone resorption and help the body maintain its bone density. Ipriflavone can help to prevent osteoporosis in postmenopausal woman. It slows down the action of osteoclasts (bone-eroding cells) allowing the osteoblasts (bone=building cells) to build up bone mass.
- **Dong Quai Root:** This is an herb that is closely related to celery. Dong Quai can help with menstrual disorders such as cessation of menstruation, pain that accompanies menstruation including headaches that are common with dysmenorreha. Dong Quai has also been shown to help postmenopausal symptoms of dryness and hot flashes.
- **Soy Isoflavone:** These are naturally present in the soybean. Research has shown that soy isoflavone can ease postmenopausal symptoms such as hot flashes, while increasing bone density. Also important for menopausal woman, soy has been shown to increase cardiovascular health by inhibiting the growth of the cells that form artery-causing plaque.
- **Black Cohosh:** This is a member of the buttercup family. Black Cohosh has been shown to effectively relieve the menopausal symptoms of hot flashes. **Woman Hormone Support Formula is recommended to postmenopausal woman and woman who suffer from dysmenorreha (painful menstruation). For postmenopausal take 1-2 caps in the morning with a meal. For woman with menstrual disorders take 1-2 caps as needed for the symptoms do not take daily. Avoid this supplement if you have a history of breast cancer or taking blood thinners.**

9. **Men's Hormone Support Formula:** This is one of the most complete formulas created for men to maintain their sexual health and youthful exuberance. This formula helps males to naturally maintain healthy testosterone levels. Testosterone is the key to maintain muscle and healthy Biomarkers. The Men's Hormone Support Formula also contains ingredients that increase blood flow, which is the key for strong erections and cardiovascular health. The Men's Hormone Support Formula contains ingredients to protect the prostate making it a complete male formula.

- **Pantothenic Acid:** This is a water-soluble vitamin, B-5. Pantothenic acid is required to sustain life making it an essential nutrient. Pantothenic Acid is needed to form coenzyme-A (CoA), which is critical for the metabolism and synthesis of carbohydrates, fats and proteins.
- **Zinc, Magnesium Aspartate (ZMA):** Testosterone is the key hormone that keeps us males young and enthusiastic to live life. Zinc is critical for testosterone production. When you combine zinc and magnesium aspartate (ZMA) it has been shown to naturally increase anabolic hormones levels, including free testosterone and IGF-1 (a key for growth hormone). ZMA helps the body to recuperate from stress and replenish its natural hormone levels.
- **L-Arginine:** Arginine enhances the production of nitric oxide (NO), a crucial compound that helps improve blood flow. NO is key for a healthy male sex organ response and overall cardiovascular health. In clinical studies, arginine has also been found to significantly raise growth hormone levels. Research data show notable strength and muscle improvement in subjects who exercised, which improves the Biomarkers and decreases fat.
- **Muira Puama:** This is a small Brazilian tree that grows across the Amazon River basin. Muira Puama has longed been used as an aphrodisiac. It has been shown to increase sexual function and is also know as "Potency Wood".
- **Avena Sativa:** Is a scientific name for a grass commonly known as oats. Avena Sativa extract has been shown to free up bound testosterone in the blood making it more bioavailable for use in the body. Avena Sativa has also been used as an erection enhancer to increase sexual performance.
- **Tribulus Terrestris Extract:** Tribulus enhances the release of luteinizing hormone (LH), which stimulates the testes to produce more testosterone. Tribulus, otherwise known as puncturevine, is an herb that has an active ingredient called protodiosein. Studies have shown that this ingredient prompts the brain to release more LH thus naturally increasing testosterone. Testosterone the key hormone to promote muscle gains and fat loss.
- **Saw Palmetto:** This supplement is used popularly in Europe for symptoms associated with an enlarged prostate. Saw Palmetto has shown multiple mechanisms of actions. It appears to possess 5-a-

reductase inhibitor activity, preventing the conversion of testosterone to dihydrotesterone (DHT). Saw Palmetto has also been shown to have anti-inflammatory properties. **Men's Hormone Support Formula is recommended for men in the Third Cycle of Health (Ages 45 years and older). It is also a great formula for hard training athletes looking for better recuperation. This formula should not be used if there is a history of prostate cancer. Recommended dosage is 2-4 caps before bed.**

10. **Corti-Lean Formula:** It is a complete stress management formula that gives you adrenal support. Corti-Lean Formula helps the body to handle and recuperate from stress. I use this formula for anyone with symptoms of an unbalanced Stress Response.

- **Ashwaganda Root:** Ashwaganda contains flavonoids and many active ingredients that aid general health. Several studies over the past few years have indicated that ashwaganda has anti-inflammatory, anti-stress, antioxidant, mind boosting and rejuvenating properties.
- **N-Acetyl-L-Carnitine:** Many nutrients have been studied for their potential in supporting brain health in older adults. N-Acetyl-L-Carntine is one of those nutrients. N-Acetyl-L-Carnitine protects neurons from oxidative stress. It also benefits mitochondrial efficiency and functions as an antioxidant within the mitochondria, helping neurons maintain optimal energy levels.
- **Siberian Ginseng Root:** Has been used for centuries in Eastern countries, including China and Russia. Siberian Ginseng is prized for its ability to restore vigor, increase longevity, enhance overall health, and stimulate memory. In Russia Siberian Ginseng has been used to help the body adapt to stressful conditions and to enhance productivity.
- **Rhodiola:** This plant has a history of medicinal use dating back to ancient Greece. Rhodiola is also known as arctic rose, it has been shown to increase the body's resistance to a variety of stress, such as chemical, biological and physical stressors. Rhodiola has been shown to prevent a drop in critical hormones such as IGF-1, dopamine and thyroid hormones and blunts the catabolic hormone cortisol.
- **Phosphatidylserine (PS):** This is a fatty chemical (phospholipids) found in cell membranes and nervous tissue and primarily maintains cell structure and function. PS is made mainly from soybeans. Research

shows PS can significantly lower levels of adrenocorticotropin hormones and cortisol, elevated during prolonged periods of stress. PS has been especially effective at improving mental function and promoting feeling of well-being. **Corti-Lean Formula can benefit the health of anyone who has high stress in his or her life. For those in the Second Cycle of Health 35 years of age and above can benefit from this formula. Recommended dose 1 cap in the a.m. with breakfast and 1-2 caps p.m. with dinner.**

11. **Better Sleep Formula:** This is a wonderful formula for anyone who is having trouble sleeping and/or cannot relax. When the Stress Response is out of balance the body will have trouble relaxing and your natural sleep patterns will be disrupted. The Better Sleep Formula allows the body and nervous system to relax naturally so you can get a deep REM sleep and wake up refreshed in the morning.

- **Magnesium:** This is a naturally occurring mineral in the body. Magnesium is important for many systems in the body, especially for the muscles, nerves, bones and the heart.
- **Valerian:** Valerian has been used as a medicinal herb since at least the times of ancient Greece and Rome. Its therapeutic uses were to treat nervousness, trembling, headaches and insomnia. Valerian helps the body to relax naturally.
- **Inositol:** This is a naturally occurring nutrient classified as a carbocyclic polyol. In the human body, inositol plays a major role in preventing fats in the liver. Inositol also aids in efficient processing of nutrients into the conversion of energy, which in turn helps the body maintain a healthy metabolism. A healthy metabolism is crucial for balancing the Stress Response. One of the main reasons inositol is in the Sleep Formula; it's considered a brain food, as it is a necessary nutrient to properly nourish the brain.
- **Melatonin:** Melatonin is a hormone produced in the pineal gland, a small gland in the brain that helps regulate our body's internal clock. Melatonin is essential to regulate our circadian rhythm (our natural cycle of sleep and waking hours). Natural melatonin levels decline gradually with age. Some adults produce very little melatonin or none at all. Without adequate melatonin the body cannot rest properly. Melatonin has also been shown to strengthen the immune system. **The Better Sleep Formula should be taken 30 minutes before**

going to bed. It can be used by anyone who is having trouble sleeping. I recommend clients in the Third Cycle of Health and above to use it daily. You should never combine this formula with any type of sleeping medication. Talk to your doctor if you are taking any anti-depressant medication.

12. **Selenium:** This is a key component of glutathione peroxidase, a major cellular antioxidant. Selenium is also an important factor for proper thyroid metabolism, it helps the conversion of T-4 to T-3 which is five times more active than T-4. A proper thyroid metabolism helps limit damage to muscles and other tissues and is an absolute key for fat burning. Research also indicates that selenium may even posses some anti-cancer properties. **I recommend selenium to anyone taking thyroid medications or a family history of thyroid disease. It's a great preventative supplement that can increase your overall health, specially for those in the Second Cycle of Health and beyond. Take 1-2 caps daily with food.**

13. **Ultra Complete Multi Vitamin Multi Mineral:** This is a supplement that is designed for Stress Response management. The Ultra Complete Multi Vitamin Multi Mineral helps eliminate the possibility of nutritional deficiencies that are often brought on by stress and nutritional quality of the diet consumed. Many of these nutrients frequently can't be produced in the body at sufficient rates to maintain optimal metabolism. **I recommend the Ultra Complete Multi Vitamin Multi Mineral for everybody. Over the years I have had great success using this supplement in combination with the Stress Management Formula. I have the client take the Stress Management Formula at breakfast and the Ultra Complete Multi Vitamin Multi Mineral formula with dinner. This combination works well in keeping the body balanced with the proper nutrients needed to balance the Stress Response.**

14. **Dehydroepiandrosterone (DHEA):** DHEA is produced by the adrenal glands and is involved in several important physiological processes in the body. These include supporting insulin function, increasing bone density, promoting mental health and it is a precursor for our sex hormones. DHEA is crucial for managing the Stress Response. DHEA helps reduce body fat, particularly from the midsection; it also increases levels IGF-1 which is important to maintain healthy growth hormone levels which is a key factor in slowing the aging process and maintaining muscle (Ten Biomarkers). DHEA levels can start to decline

in the early 20s in individuals who have high stress levels. **DHEA has been a little controversial over the last few years. I have personally seen drastic changes for the better in client's health once they start supplementing DHEA. With that being said, I recommend that clients get a simple blood test (see appendix B) to see if they are within optimal ranges. Elevated DHEA can throw the other hormones in the body out of balance causing weight gain, anger, fatigue and facial hair. Recommended dosage 25-50 milligrams for men and 10-25 milligrams for woman. I recommend testing DHEA levels before and after taking the supplement. Do not take DHEA if you have any history of cancer and consult your physician first.**

BioFit Supplements can be ordered at: www.biofitprogram.com

Bibliography

- Cannon Walter (1929) Bodily Changes in Pain, Hunger, Fear and r age. New york-Appleton.
- Tsigos, C and Chrousus, G.P. (2002) Hypothalam ic-pituitary-Adrenal axis-neroendocrine factors and stress. Journal of Psycholosomatic research, 53, 865, 871.
- Tiidus, Peter, M.—Skeletal Muscle damage and repair, human Kinetics, 2008, Pg.137 "Alterations in Glucose Transport."
- Inflammation, Heart Diseaseand Stroke: The Role of C-reactive Protein." American Heart Association, August 3rd, 2009. http://www.americanheart.org.
- Evans, William, Ph.D.,Rosenberg, Irwin H. MD-Biomarkers: The 10 Keys to prolonging vitality. New York, New york 10020,Fireside,1992
- Hansen, Carolyn. Sarcopenia—on't let this happen to you", 2009-02-20 http://www.articlesphere.com/Article/Sarcopenia.
- Sears, Barry Dr. "Anti-Infalmmation Zone: reversing the silent epidemic that is destroying our health. Harper Collins, 2005
- Chopra, Deepak. "Ageless Body, Timeless Mind." Three Rivers Press. 1998.
- Campbell, Neil A.; Brad Williamson; Robin J. Heyden. "Biology: Exploring Life" Boston, massachussetts, Pearson, Prentice hall, 2006.
- Andrews, Zane, Dr "Killer Carbs: Scientist finds keys to overeating as we age" Science Daily, 2008.
- Kimball C, Murlin J. Aqueous extracts of pancreas, some precipitation reactions of insulin. J Biol Chem 1923;58: 337-348.
- Minton, Barbara; Hormones part III: Optimal levels of cortisol, insulin and thyroid are essential to vibrant health: Sources; 4221 Reis, MD/Ob-Gyn, natural hormone balance for women; T.S. Wiley Lights out, Sabre sciences; about hormones; Herb Slavin, MD, Phillip Lee MIller, MD

and Gordon Reynolds, MD Suzanne Summers, break through: Natural news.com Jan 13, 2009

- Spiegel K, Leproult R, Van Cauter E. "Impact of sleep debt on metabolic and endocrine function. Lancer 1999; 354, 1435-39.
- University of Connecticut school of medicine in Farmington, USA, Altern ther. health Med. 2009 may-june; 15 93):44-52 PMID:19472664
- Coleman M. Andrew, "A dictionary of phsychology" London, kings college, Oxford University Press, 2006.
- American Sports Data INC; The latest statistics on America's obesity epidemic. http://americansportsdata.com/obesitystats.asp, 2004
- Weinsier, R.L.; Do adaptive changes in metabolic rate favor weight regain in weight-reduced individuals? An examination of the fat set point theory; The American Journal of Clincal Nutrition, 72(5)1088, (2000)
- Blundell, J.E.; Regulation of appetite: Rule of leptin in signaling systems for drive and satiety: International journal of obesity and related metabolic disorders 25(1), 529. (2001)
- Medicinenet.com; Definition of adiponectin http://www.medterms.com/(2004)
- Murphy, K.G. Bloom, S.R. "Gut hormones in the control of appetite: Experimental physciooogy, 89, 507-516 (2004)

Index

CPSIA information can be obtained at www.ICGtesting.com
Printed in the USA
LVOW121925270213

321847LV00001B/1/P